The Ulcerative Colitis Cookbook

Easy and Delicious Meals for the Next 18 Months to Boost Your Digestive Health | Contains a 28-day meal plan to improve health for those with IBD.

Author

Willie B. Robinson

Table of Content

Introduction

Every year, an estimated half a million new cases of ulcerative colitis are diagnosed. Five million Americans have this disease. Peptic ulcer disease is The most frequently affecting persons born in the mid-twentieth century. Ulcer disease prevalence rises with age, peaking between 55 and 65. 35% of gastric ulcer patients develop complications, and duodenal ulcers are more common in men than women.. Although peptic ulcer disease is not fatal, it causes significant suffering and expense.

This cookbook is intended to assist those recently diagnosed with an ulcer. Making dietary options after being diagnosed with ulcer disease for the first time might be difficult. Use this recipe carefully if you want to achieve it regardless of your circumstances. Thanks to a 28-day meal plan and 120 tasty and healthful meals, you may eat and prepare with pride.

Numerous research studies have associated dietary changes as potential treatments for stomach ulcers. Anyone suffering from an ulcer should adhere to the ulcer diet. Peptic ulcers, also known as stomach ulcers, are painful digestive tract sores. It can treat gastritis and gastrointestinal issues. Although medicine is more likely to be part of your ulcer treatment strategy than food, adding dietary adjustments may expedite your healing and lower the probability of recurrence.

Adhering to an ulcer diet and other treatment suggestions may help ease symptom-inducing nutritional deficits and facilitate recovery. If you have Crohn's disease, bacterial infections, or celiac disease, avoiding foods that irritate your stomach and small intestine may help reduce your ulcer symptoms.

What is Ulcerative Colitis?

Every year, an estimated half a million new cases of ulcerative colitis are diagnosed. Five million Americans have this disease. Peptic ulcer disease is The most frequently affecting persons born in the mid-twentieth century. Ulcer disease prevalence rises with age, peaking between 55 and 65. 35% of gastric ulcer patients develop complications, and duodenal ulcers are more common in men than women.. Although peptic ulcer disease is not fatal, it causes significant suffering and expense.

This cookbook is intended to assist those recently diagnosed with an ulcer. Making dietary options after being diagnosed with ulcer disease for the first time might be difficult. Use this recipe carefully if you want to achieve it regardless of your circumstances. Thanks to a 28-day meal plan and 120 tasty and healthful meals, you may eat and prepare with pride.

Numerous research studies have associated dietary changes as potential treatments for stomach ulcers. Anyone suffering from an ulcer should adhere to the ulcer diet. Peptic ulcers, also known as stomach ulcers, are painful digestive tract sores. It can treat gastritis and gastrointestinal issues. Although medicine is more likely to be part of your ulcer treatment strategy than food, adding dietary adjustments may expedite your healing and lower the probability of recurrence.

Adhering to an ulcer diet and other treatment suggestions may ease symptom-inducing nutritional deficits and facilitate recovery. If you have Crohn's disease, bacterial infections, or celiac disease, avoiding foods that irritate your stomach and small intestine may help reduce your ulcer symptoms.

Causes of Ulcerative Colitis

Though the specific etiology of ulcerative colitis is unknown, it is assumed to be caused by genetic, environmental, and immunological factors.

Ulcerative colitis runs in families, a study found. It is not a genetic condition; other factors are most likely at work.

Environmental variables include smoking, eating a high-fat or refined-sugar diet, and being exposed to certain viruses or bacteria, all of which increase the chance of developing ulcerative colitis.

Immunological factors: It is believed that an aberrant immunological response in the colon causes ulcerative colitis. The immune system defends the body from hazardous microorganisms in healthy humans. Even so, in those with ulcerative colitis, the immune system wrongly assaults the colon lining, causing inflammation and ulceration.

Although stress and emotional factors do not directly cause ulcerative colitis, they can exacerbate symptoms in some people.

While these variables may increase your chances of developing ulcerative colitis, they do not necessarily cause it. Furthermore, some persons may develop ulcerative colitis without identifying risk factors.

Symptoms Of Ulcerative Colitis

From mild to severe, ulcerative colitis symptoms can differ from person to person. The following are some typical signs of ulcerative colitis:

- ❖ Abdominal pain and cramping
- ❖ Diarrhoea, which may be bloody
- ❖ Rectal bleeding
- ❖ The urgency to have a bowel movement
- ❖ Inability to have a bowel movement despite the urgency
- ❖ Weight loss
- ❖ Fatigue and weakness
- ❖ Loss of appetite
- ❖ Anaemia
- ❖ Joint pain and swelling
- ❖ Skin rashes

The person's symptoms can change, and there might be times when they are minimal to nonexistent and in remission. These remissions, though, might be followed by episodes where symptoms worsen. When you notice these symptoms, you should consult a doctor because ulcerative colitis can cause life-threatening side effects if not treated.

Chapter 1:- Breakfast Recipe

1.Sausage and Egg Breakfast Sandwich

Ingredients:

- 4 English muffins, split and toasted
- Eight breakfast sausage patties
- Four slices of cheddar cheese
- Four large eggs
- Salt and pepper, to taste
- 2 tbsp. Butter or oil

Instructions:

1. In a big pan over medium-high heat, fry and brown the morning sausage patties.
2. Remove the sausage patties from the skillet and place them on a dish.
3. Melt the butter or heat the oil in the same pan over medium heat.
4. Cook for two to three minutes after the whites are set but the yolks are still runny in the skillet.
5. Prepare eggs to taste with salt and pepper.
6. Put a pork patty on each English muffin bottom before making sandwiches.
7. On top of the sausage patty, sprinkle some cheddar cheese and a fried egg.
8. Place the top half of the English muffin on top of the egg.
9. Hot egg-and-meat breakfast sandwiches.

2.Classic Eggs Benedict

Ingredients:

- 4 English muffins, split and toasted
- Eight slices of Canadian bacon
- Four large eggs
- 1/2 cups of unsalted butter
- Three egg yolks
- 1 tbsp. fresh lemon juice
- 1/4 tsp. salt
- Pinch of cayenne pepper

Instructions:

1. The Canadian bacon should be lightly cooked in a pan on both sides. Stay warm.
2. A large pot should be filled with two inches of water, then simmered.
3. Egg yolks, lemon juice, salt, and cayenne pepper in a medium bowl.
4. Butter should bubble in a small saucepan over medium heat.
5. The egg yolk mixture should be whisked continually while being set over hot water until it thickens and doubles in volume.
6. Whisk in melted butter gradually until the sauce is thick and creamy.
7. You may poach eggs so that the whites are solid, but the yolks are still fluid by cracking the eggs into the simmering water and cooking them for 3–4 minutes.

8. Assemble two toasted English muffin halves on a plate. Each half is topped with a poached egg, Canadian bacon, and hollandaise sauce. Serve immediately.

3.French Toast

Ingredients:
- Four slices of bread
- Two eggs
- 1/4 cups of milk
- 1 tbsp. sugar
- 1 tsp. vanilla extract
- 1/4 tsp. ground cinnamon
- Butter or oil for cooking
- Powdered sugar and maple syrup for serving

Instructions:
1. Combine the eggs, milk, sugar, vanilla extract, and ground cinnamon in a shallow bowl.
2. Coat both sides When dipping each bread slice in the egg mixture.
3. A nonstick pan that is already hot should get a modest amount of butter or oil.
4. Once the butter has melted or the oil is hot, add the bread slices to the skillet and fry for 2-3 minutes on each side or until golden brown.
5. Continue with the remaining bread slices.
6. After serving, powdered sugar and maple syrup should be added to hot French toast.

4.Breakfast Burrito

Ingredients:

- Four large flour tortillas
- Six large eggs
- 1/4 cups of milk
- Salt and pepper, to taste
- 1 tbsp. butter or oil
- 1/2 cups of shredded cheddar cheese
- Four slices of cooked bacon, chop
- 1/4 cups of chop fresh cilantro
- Salsa and sour cream for serving

Instructions:

1. Combine the eggs, milk, salt, and pepper in a large dish.
2. A sizable pan that is already heated should be put in the butter or oil.
3. After the butter or oil melts, add the egg mixture to the skillet and stir constantly until the eggs are scrambled and cooked.
4. Oven or microwave the tortillas. To make burritos, place a tortilla on a tray and top with scrambled eggs, cheddar cheese, chopped bacon, and fresh cilantro.
5. Rolling the tortilla properly involves tucking the ends in as you go.
6. Continue when there are leftover toppings and tortillas.
7. Salsa, sour cream, and hot breakfast sandwiches should be offered on the side.

5. Quiche Lorraine

Ingredients:

- One pie crust (store-bought or homemade)
- Eight slices of bacon, chop
- One small onion, chop
- Four large eggs
- 1 cups of heavy cream
- 1/2 tsp. salt
- 1/4 tsp. black pepper
- 1/8 tsp. ground nutmeg
- 1 1/2 cups of shredded Swiss cheese

Instructions:

1. The oven should be preheated at 375°F (190°C).
2. Fill a 9-inch pie plate with pie dough. After cutting the edges, store them.
3. In a skillet over medium heat, crisp up the diced bacon. After using the skillet, remove it and drain on paper towels.
4. Sauté the chopped onion in the same pan until tender and translucent. Dry it.
5. Eggs, heavy cream, salt, pepper, and ground nutmeg in a medium bowl.
6. Spread the cooked bacon and sautéed onion evenly over the pie crust's bottom.
7. Spread the Swiss cheese on top of the bacon and onion.
8. Pour egg mixture over cheese.
9. In a preheated oven, bake the quiche for 35 to 40 minutes until the filling is firm and the top is brown.
10. Before serving, let the quiche rest.

6. Yogurt Parfait with Granola and Fruit

Ingredients:

- 2 cups of Greek yogurt
- 1/4 cups of honey
- 1 tsp. vanilla extract
- 2 cups of mixed berries, sliced or chopped
- 2 cups of granola

Instructions:

1. Combine Greek yogurt, honey, and vanilla extract in a bowl.
2. Serve the yogurt mixture in four bowls or cups of after dividing it in half.
3. On top of the yogurt, spread a layer of oats and mixed fruit.
4. Layering continues, and cereal is the final layer.
5. Yogurt parfaits can be served right away or after being chilled and covered.

7. Delicious Egg Salad for Sandwiches

Ingredients:

- Eight eggs
- ½ cups of mayonnaise
- ¼ cups of chopped green onion
- 1 tsp. prepared yellow mustard
- ¼ tsp. paprika
- salt and pepper to taste

Instructions:

1. The eggs and cool water should be combined in a saucepan. Turn off the heat when water boils quickly. Boil eggs covered for 10–12 minutes. After being taken out of the cooking water, peel, cut, and allow to cool.

2. Combine the chopped eggs, mayonnaise, mustard, and green onion in a bowl. Season with salt, pepper, and paprika. After stirring, plate with your favorite bread or biscuits.

8.Scrambled Egg Muffin Cups of

Ingredients:

- ½ lb bulk pork sausage
- 12 eggs
- ½ cups of chop onion
- ½ cups of chopped green bell pepper, or to taste
- ½ tsp. salt
- ¼ tsp. ground black pepper
- ¼ tsp. garlic powder
- ½ cups of shredded Cheddar cheese

Instructions:

1. Three hundred fifty degrees Fahrenheit (175 degrees C) in the oven. You should lightly oil or line twelve muffin pans with paper liners.

2. Heat a large skillet over medium-high heat. Once added, the sausage is cooked for 10 to 15 minutes or until it is uniformly browned, crumbly, and no longer pink. Take the oil out.

3. The eggs should be beaten in a big dish. Salt, garlic powder, onion, and green pepper should be added. Cheese complements pork. Spoon batter into muffin tins.
4. 20–25 minutes of baking should clean a knife inserted near the center.

9.Blueberry Pancakes

Ingredients:
- 1 1/2 cups of all-purpose flour
- 2 tbsp. sugar
- 2 tsp. baking powder
- 1/2 tsp. baking soda
- 1/4 tsp. salt
- 1 1/4 cups of milk
- Two large eggs
- 2 tbsp. melted butter or oil
- 1 cups of fresh blueberries
- Butter and maple syrup for serving

Instructions:
1. Combine the flour, sugar, baking soda, baking powder, and salt
2. in a large bowl.
3. Combine the milk, eggs, and melted butter or oil in another bowl.
4. Mix the dry ingredients first, then the wet. Do not over-mix the dough; a few lumps are acceptable.
5. Slowly incorporate the strawberries.

6. Heat a large pan or grill to a medium-high temperature. In the pan, the butter needs to be melted.
7. A 1/4 cups of measuring cups of should be used to pour the mixture onto the skillet.
8. After two to three minutes of frying the pancakes on the first side, the edges should be firm, and the top should be bubbly.
9. When the second side is golden brown, flip the pancakes over and cook them for an additional 1 to 2 minutes.
10.   It is time to serve warm blueberry crepes with butter and maple syrup.

10.   Super Easy Egg Casserole

Ingredients:
- Six eggs, whisked
- 1 cups of shredded Cheddar cheese
- Six slices bacon diced
- Two slices of bread cubed
- ⅓ red bell pepper, diced
- Two green onions, chop
- 3 tbsp. milk
- ½ tsp. garlic, either chopped or to taste
- Black pepper and salt to taste.

Instructions:
1. 350 °F (175 degrees C) in the oven. Grease a pastry pan measuring 9 x 13 inches.
2. Before pouring into the baking dish, mix the eggs, cheese, bacon, bread, red bell pepper, green onion, milk, garlic, salt, and black pepper in a bowl.

3. In a preheated oven, bake eggs for 20–25 minutes until done.

11.   Spinach and Feta Omelette

Ingredients:
- Four large eggs
- 1/4 cups of milk or cream
- Salt and pepper, to taste
- 1 tbsp. butter or oil
- 1 cups of fresh spinach leaves, chop
- 1/4 cups of crumbled feta cheese

Instructions:
1. In a small bowl, combine the eggs, milk or cream, salt, and pepper.
2. In a small nonstick pan, the butter or oil should be warmed over medium heat.
3. Once the butter has melted or the oil is heated, add the chopped spinach to the pan and cook for 1-2 minutes or until wilted.
4. Pour the egg mixture onto the skillet, then use a spatula to gently lift the edges of the omelet to let the uncooked egg flow below.
5. Once the eggs are mostly set, top one side of the omelet with the crumbled feta cheese.
6. Flip the omelet over the cheese with a spatula.
7. Once the cheese has melted, cook the eggs for an additional 1-2 minutes or until they are cooked to your liking.
8. Slide the hot omelet to a dish and set it down.

12.   Basted Eggs

Ingredients:

- 1 ½ tbsp. salted butter
- Two large eggs
- 1 tbsp. Water
- ⅛ tsp. freshly ground black pepper
- One pinch of flaky sea salt, or to taste

Instructions:

1. Melt butter in a nonstick skillet over medium heat. Carefully crack the eggs into the skillet and cook for about a minute until the yolks are almost set. When the whites are done but the yolks are still liquid, add water, cover the pan, lower the heat to medium, and simmer for 1–2 minutes. The cover is removed, and the eggs are transferred to a serving plate. Add some cracked pepper and flaky salt as a garnish if you'd like. Serve immediately.

13.   Bacon and Egg Breakfast Pizza

Ingredients:

- 1 lb pizza dough
- 1/2 cups of tomato sauce
- 1 cups of shredded mozzarella cheese
- Four slices bacon, cooked and crumbled
- Four large eggs
- Salt and pepper, to taste
- 1 tbsp. Chop fresh parsley

Instructions:

1. The oven should be heated to 425°F (220°C).
2. Stretch pizza dough to a 12-inch circle on lightly floured surface.
3. Place pizza dough on a parchment-lined baking sheet.
4. Spread tomato sauce on pizza crust, leaving a 1-inch border.
5. Add the grated mozzarella cheese and bacon bits to the tomato sauce.
6. The eggs should be evenly spaced out on the pie.
7. Prepare eggs to taste with salt and pepper.
8. The dough should be golden and the eggs cooked after 12–15 minutes.
9. Spread the parsley on top of the pizza if you'd like.
10. Pizza for breakfast should be served hot and in pieces.

14. Fluffy French Toast

Ingredients:

- ¼ cups of all-purpose flour
- 1 cups of milk
- Three eggs
- 1 tbsp. white sugar
- 1 tsp. vanilla extract
- ½ tsp. ground cinnamon
- 1 pinch salt
- 12 thick slices of bread

Instructions:

1. Fill a large mixing bowl with flour. Gradually whisk in the milk. Salt, cinnamon, sugar, vanilla extract, and eggs should all be well combined.
2. Bake the pizza until the dough is golden and the eggs are done.
3. The milk mixture should completely cover the bread pieces.
4. Cook the bread in batches on the skillet until golden brown on both sides. Serve hot.

15. Banana Bread

Ingredients:

- 2 cups of all-purpose flour
- 1 tsp. baking soda
- 1/4 tsp. salt
- 1/2 cups of unsalted butter, softened
- 3/4 cups of brown sugar
- Two large eggs, beaten
- Three ripe bananas, mashed
- 1/2 cups of plain Greek yogurt
- 1 tsp. vanilla extract

Instructions:

1. Preheat the oven to 350 degrees Fahrenheit (175 degrees Celsius). Spray a 9x5-inch loaf pan.
2. Flour, baking soda, and salt in a medium bowl.
3. Cream the butter and brown sugar together in a separate, large mixing bowl until fluffy.

4. Greek yogurt, eggs, mashed bananas, and vanilla extract are just some of the ingredients that need to be thoroughly mixed together.
5. Gradually mix in the dry ingredients until they are fully incorporated.
6. Fill the greased loaf pan with the batter.
7. After 60–65 minutes, a toothpick should come out clean from the bread's center.
8. After 10 minutes, move the banana bread to a wire rack to cool completely.
9. The banana bread should be served warm or, at room temperature, sliced.

16.   Basic Biscuits

Ingredients:
- 2 cups of all-purpose flour
- 1 tbsp. baking powder
- ½ tsp. salt
- ½ cups of shortening
- ¾ cups of cold milk

Instructions:
1. Prepare the ingredients, then preheat the oven to 450°F (230°C).
2. Sift flour, baking soda, and salt in a large bowl. Fork or pastry blender the shortening into coarse crumbs.
3. Fork-whisk the milk into the flour mixture. When the dough is moist and pliable and starting to pull away from the edge of the bowl, add milk and continue to stir.

4. On a lightly floured surface, quickly knead the dough 5–7 times.
5. Roll the dough into a 1/2-inch sheet and cut biscuits with a floured cookie cutter. Repeat the rolling and cutting steps while pushing any remaining dough together.
6. Bake cookies on ungreased baking sheets for 10 minutes until golden brown.

17.   Breakfast Quesadilla

Ingredients:
- Two large flour tortillas
- Four large eggs, beaten
- 1/2 cups of cooked and crumbled breakfast sausage
- 1/2 cups of shredded cheddar cheese
- 1/4 cups of chopped green onions
- Salt and pepper, to taste
- 1 tbsp. vegetable oil

Instructions:
1. A giant skillet should be heated to medium.
2. Salt and pepper the eggs in a mixing bowl.
3. Salt and beat eggs in a bowl.Heat the breakfast meat for 3–4 minutes until it's browned and crumbled.
4. Add the beaten eggs to the pan and scramble them for 3 to 4 minutes or until fully cooked.
5. The eggs and sausage should be transferred to a dish after turning off the heat in the skillet.
6. Make use of paper cloth to clean the skillet.

7. A flour tortilla should be placed in the skillet with half the shredded cheddar cheese on one side.
8. Top the meat and scrambled eggs with half the cheese.
9. Sprinkle half the chopped green onions over the eggs and pork.
10. To form a half-moon, fold the remaining tortilla over the center.
11. Repeat with the remaining components and tortillas.
12. Over medium heat, add the vegetable oil to the pan.
13. Cook the quesadillas for 2–3 minutes per side until the cheese melts and the tortillas are crunchy.
14. To serve, take the quesadillas out of the skillet and cut them into pieces.

18. Breakfast Hash with Sweet Potatoes and Sausage

Ingredients:
- 1 lb sweet potatoes, peeled and diced
- 1 lb breakfast sausage, casings removed
- One red bell pepper, diced
- One yellow onion, diced
- 1 tsp. dried thyme
- 1/2 tsp. smoked paprika
- Salt and pepper, to taste
- 2 tbsp. olive oil
- Four large eggs

Instructions:

1. The oven should be set to 400°F (200°C).
2. Combine the diced sweet potatoes in a big dish with the red bell pepper, yellow onion, dried thyme, smoky paprika, salt, and pepper.
3. Layer the vegetable mixture on a baking sheet.
4. 20–25 minutes in the oven caramelizes sweet potatoes.
5. While the vegetables are roasting, preheat a sizable skillet over medium-high heat.
6. Breakfast sausage should be added to the skillet and cooked for 8 to 10 minutes or until it is browned and crumbled.
7. After cooking the vegetables, add them to the skillet with the sausage and toss.
8. Crack an egg into each of the four hash mixture wells you make.
9. Cook the eggs for 5-7 minutes in a covered pan to your liking.
10. Serve hot.

19.   Greek Yogurt Waffles

Ingredients:

- 2 cups of all-purpose flour
- 2 tsp. baking powder
- 1/2 tsp. baking soda
- 1/2 tsp. salt
- 2 tbsp. granulated sugar
- 1 3/4 cups of milk
- 1/2 cups of plain Greek yogurt
- Two large eggs

- 1/4 cups of unsalted butter, melted
- 1 tsp. vanilla extract

Instructions:

1. Prepare your pancake maker.
2. Mix the sugar, salt, baking powder, and soda, and flour together in a large bowl.
3. Combine the milk, Greek yogurt, eggs, melted butter, and vanilla extract in a different mixing bowl.
4. Stir the batter until it is smooth after incorporating the wet ingredients into the dry ones.
5. Scoop the batter onto the waffle iron by the manufacturer's instructions for the recommended batter quantity and cooking time.
6. To use up the last of the dough, continue.
7. You are presenting the waffles hot with your choice of toppings, such as fresh fruit, whipped cream, or maple syrup.

20.   Biscuits and Gravy

Ingredients:
For the biscuits:

- 2 cups of all-purpose flour
- 2 tsp. baking powder
- 1/2 tsp. baking soda
- 1/2 tsp. salt
- 1/2 cups of unsalted butter, chilled and cubed
- 3/4 cups of buttermilk

For the sausage gravy:

- 1 lb breakfast sausage
- 1/3 cups of all-purpose flour
- 3 cups of whole milk
- Salt and pepper, to taste

Instructions:

1. The oven should be heated to 425°F (220°C).
2. In a large bowl, whisk together the flour, baking powder, salt, and baking soda.
3. Combine the flour mixture with the cooled butter with a pastry blender or your hands until it resembles coarse crumbs.
4. Stir in the buttermilk while adding it to the dish until the dough comes together.
5. Now, transfer the dough to a floured surface and knead it several times until it is smooth and elastic.
6. Roll out the dough to a 1-inch thickness, then cut out the biscuits using a glass or a biscuit cutter.
7. Place cookies on a baking sheet lined with parchment paper.
8. If you want golden cookies, bake them for 12-15 minutes.
9. While baking the biscuits, cook the morning sausage for 8 to 10 minutes, or until it is browned and crumbled, in a big skillet over medium heat.
10. The meat should be blended with the flour after being added.
11. As you gradually pour in the milk, cook the gravy for 5 to 7 minutes while stirring continually.
12. When making the gravy, season with salt and pepper for flavor.
13. Serve the warmed biscuits with the pig gravy on top.

21.   Oatmeal Soda Bread

Ingredients:

- 3 ½ cups of all-purpose flour
- ½ cups of quick cooking oats
- 1 tsp. salt
- 1 tsp. baking powder
- 1 tsp. baking soda
- 1 (8 oz.) container of low-fat sour cream
- ¾ cups of skim milk
- 2 tbsp. honey
- 1 tbsp. white sugar
- ¼ cups of melted butter
- 2 tbsp. butter melted

Instructions:

1. The oven should be set to 375 degrees. 190 degrees Celsius.
2. Flour, 1/2 cup oats, salt, baking soda, and baking powder should be mixed together in a sizable bowl.
3. Mix the milk, honey, sugar, and sour cream in another bowl. Stir just long enough to incorporate the addition into the flour mixture. Stir in the softened butter or margarine.
4. Roll out the dough on a baking sheet coated with cooking spray. Create a light-mounded circle with a circumference of roughly 8 inches. Brush the bread with melted butter or margarine, then top with the last spoonful of oats. Use a knife to cut the top of the bread into pieces.
5. Caramelization should occur after about 40 minutes in the oven. Only cut when the cooling process is finished.

22. Ham and Cheese Breakfast Casserole

Ingredients:

- Six large eggs
- 2 cups of milk
- 1 tsp. ground mustard
- 1/2 tsp. salt
- 1/4 tsp. black pepper
- 8 cups of cubed bread, such as French bread or sourdough
- 2 cups of shredded cheddar cheese
- 1 cups of diced ham
- 1/4 cups of chopped green onions

Instructions:

1. Set the oven's temperature to 350°F (175°C).
2. In a large bowl, thoroughly combine the eggs, milk, mustard powder, salt, and pepper.
3. Cubed bread should be added to the mixing dish and stirred to distribute the egg mixture evenly.
4. Mix the shredded cheddar cheese, diced ham, and green onions in a mixing dish.
5. Put the ingredients into a 9-by-13-inch baking dish that has been greased.
6. When the eggs are set and the surface of the casserole is golden brown, cover the baking dish with foil and bake it for 40 to 45 minutes.
7. Remove the foil and continue baking for another 10 to 15 minutes until the cheese is melted and bubbling.
8. Before cutting and serving, allow the casserole to settle for a few minutes.

23. Shakshuka

Ingredients:

- 2 tbsp. olive oil
- One onion, diced
- Two garlic cloves minced
- One red bell pepper, diced
- One can (28 oz.) of crushed tomatoes
- 1 tsp. ground cumin
- 1/2 tsp. smoked paprika
- Salt and black pepper, to taste
- 4-6 large eggs
- Fresh parsley, chop, for garnish
- Crusty bread for serving

Instructions:

1. Olive oil should be heated in a sizable pan over medium heat.
2. To soften the onion and garlic, add them to the pan and cook for 5 to 7 minutes.
3. Cook the diced red bell pepper in the pan for 5 minutes or until it softens.
4. Coat the bottom of the pan with the oil and then add the crushed tomatoes, cumin, smoked paprika, salt, and black pepper.
5. Cook the sauce for 10 to 15 minutes, or until it reaches the desired thickness.
6. Make wells in the tomato sauce with a spoon, then drop an egg into each one.
7. Keep the skillet covered and cook for another 5 to 7 minutes, or until the egg whites are set but the yolks are still runny.

8. Dive in with some crusty bread and some minced fresh parsley.

24.   Sweet French Toast

Ingredients:
- 3 eggs
- ¼ cups of milk
- 2 ½ tbsp. maple syrup
- 1 tsp. vanilla extract
- 1 tsp. ground cinnamon
- ⅓ cups of cornflakes cereal, crumbled
- Eight slices of white bread
- 2 tbsp. Confectioners' sugar for dusting

Instructions:
1. Whisk together the eggs, milk, maple syrup, vanilla, and cinnamon in a medium bowl. Add a modest handful of crumbled cornflakes to the mixture. Thoroughly stir.
2. Bread slices should soak in the mixture for two to three minutes.
3. Warm a griddle or skillet over medium heat and lightly oil it. Placed in the pan, bread slices must be toasted on both sides. Top with confectioners' sugar and serve warm.

25. Crème Brûlée French Toast

Ingredients:

- ½ cups of unsalted butter
- 1 cups of packed brown sugar
- 2 tbsp. corn syrup
- 6 (1-inch thick) slices of French bread
- Five large eggs
- 1 ½ cups of half-and-half cream
- 1 tsp. vanilla extract
- 1 tsp. Brandy-based orange liqueur
- ¼ tsp. salt

Instructions:

1. In a small skillet set over medium heat, melt the butter. Corn syrup and brown sugar should be stirred in until the sugar is dissolved. The mixture should fill a 9x13-inch pan about halfway.
2. Bread crusts should be removed and arranged in a uniform layer in the baking dish. Simply put, you need to whisk together some eggs, milk, vanilla, bourbon, and salt. Toss into the mix. Cover and chill for 8 hours or overnight.
3. Set the oven to 350°F. (175 degrees C). In the interim, reheat the food from the fridge at room temperature.
4. Bake for 35 to 40 minutes, uncovered, in the preheated oven or until puffy and faintly browned.

26. Breakfast Strata with Sausage and Spinach

Ingredients:

- 1 lb Italian sausage, casing removed
- One onion, diced
- One red bell pepper, diced
- 2 cups of baby spinach, chop
- Eight slices of white bread, cubed
- 2 cups of shredded cheddar cheese
- Eight large eggs
- 2 cups of milk
- 1 tsp. salt
- 1/4 tsp. black pepper

Instructions:

1. 350°F (175°C) should be the oven's setting.
2. The meat must be well-cooked and browned in a sizable skillet set over medium heat. Transfer the sausage to a dish with a slotted spoon and set aside.
3. The red bell pepper and onion should be added to the same skillet and cooked for 5 to 7 minutes or until tender.
4. Cook spinach in the pan for 2–3 minutes until it wilts.
5. Spray cooking oil into a 9x13-inch baking pan.
6. Over the bread slices in the baking dish, top with the cooked sausage, prepared veggies and shredded cheddar cheese.
7. Combine the eggs, milk, salt, and pepper in a large bowl.
8. Carefully cover the bread cubes in the baking dish with the egg mixture.

9. The baking dish should be covered with foil and baked for 45 minutes.
10. When the egg mixture has set and the top is golden brown, remove the foil and bake for another 15–20 minutes.
11. The strata need a few minutes to chill before cutting and serving.

27. Irish Soda Bread

Ingredients:
- 4 cups of all-purpose flour
- 1 cups of white sugar
- 2 tsp. baking powder
- 1 tsp. baking soda
- ½ tsp. salt
- 1-pint sour cream
- 1 cups of raisins
- Three eggs

Instructions:
1. (165 degrees C) Turn the oven on at 325 degrees Fahrenheit. Grease two 8x4-inch bread pans before baking.
2. Flour, salt, baking soda, and baking powder must all be mixed. The yolks, sour cream, and raisins should just be barely mixed. Distribute the batter evenly between the pans.
3. In a hot oven, loaves should bake for an hour.

28. Muesli

Ingredients:

- 4 ½ cups of rolled oats
- 1 cups of raisins
- ½ cups of toasted wheat germ
- ½ cups of wheat bran
- ½ cups of oat bran
- ½ cups of chop walnuts
- ¼ cups of packed brown sugar
- ¼ cups of raw sunflower seeds

Instructions:

1. Mix the oats, raisins, wheat germ, wheat bran, oat bran, walnuts, brown sugar, and sunflower seeds in a sizable dish. If stored in an airtight container, muesli has a shelf life of up to two months when kept at room temperature.

29. Crescent Breakfast Squares

Ingredients:

- Two 12x16-inch parchment paper sheets
- 2 (12 oz.) packages of crescent roll dough
- Eight slices deli ham
- 2 tbsp. Dijon mustard, or more to taste
- 3 tbsp. unsalted butter, divided
- ½ cups of diced onion
- ½ cups of diced red bell pepper
- Ten large eggs
- 1 tbsp. heavy whipping cream, also known as half-and-half,

- one pinch of salt, and freshly ground black pepper to taste
- Eight slices of Swiss cheese
- 1 tbsp. bagel seasoning

Instructions:

2. The oven temperature should be set to 375°F (190°C).
3. Spread out each parchment sheet in a workspace. One can of filling is spread over each crescent-shaped piece of dough. Make sure the perforations are shut as you roll the dough into two 10x15-inch squares, one for each part of the parchment.
4. Save the second piece of dough for another time. On a 13x18-inch sheet pan, place one rectangle of dough with the parchment paper still attached.
5. Over the top of the initial layer of dough, arrange the ham slices, leaving a 1/2-inch border all around. Smear the ham slices with some Dijon mustard.
6. Melt one tablespoon in a big pan. on medium heat of the butter. After three minutes of cooking and stirring, the onions and peppers should be tender.
7. Melt one tablespoon while lowering the heat to medium. Vegetables in a skillet of butter.
8. The eggs, half-and-half or cream, salt, and pepper should all be combined thoroughly in a large dish. Pour the egg mixture over the vegetables in the pan. Elevate and move the meal with a spatula when the eggs are almost set but still seem wet.
9. Spoon the barely cooked egg mixture equally over the ham slices while preserving the 1/2-inch dough border. Swiss cheese slices should be arranged on top of the eggs.

10.   As you lay the second rectangle of dough over everything, use the paper to help you align it. With care, remove the form. After joining the corners of the two dough rectangles with damp fingertips, crimp them with a fork.

11.   Apply the last tablespoon of melted butter to the dough with a pastry brush. The flavor of a bagel should be used to season everything.

12.   Cook for 20–25 minutes in an oven that has been preheated until a beautiful browning has occurred. Remove from oven and set on a wire rack to cool for about 15 minutes. Slice the food into serving sizes with a sharp knife.

Chapter 2:- Lunch Recipes

30.   Grilled Cheese Sandwich

Ingredients:
- Four slices of white bread
- 3 tbsp. butter, divided
- Two pieces of Cheddar cheese

Instructions:
1. A nonstick pan should be preheated to medium. Butter a piece of bread liberally on one side.
2. To make a grilled cheese sandwich, heat a skillet and add one slice of cheese and the buttered side of bread.
3. A second piece of bread should be butter-side up and placed on the cheese.
4. After the bottom has browned slightly, flip it over and continue cooking until the cheese has melted.

5. Repetition is required with the remaining two pieces of bread, butter, and cheese.

31. Delicious Egg Salad for Sandwiches

Ingredients:
- Eight eggs
- ½ cups of mayonnaise
- ¼ cups of chopped green onion
- 1 tsp. prepared yellow mustard
- ¼ tsp. paprika
- salt and pepper to taste

Instructions:
1. Add the eggs to a saucepan, then the cold water. Turn off the fire once the water has come to a rolling boil.
2. Keep the eggs covered and in boiling water for 10–12 minutes. Peel, chop, and let cool after removing from the cooking water.
3. Combine the chop eggs with the mustard, mayonnaise, and green onion in a dish. Season with smoked paprika, salt, and black pepper. Mix in your favorite bread or biscuits and serve.

32. Best Cream of Broccoli Soup

Ingredients:

- 5 tbsp. butter, divided
- One onion, chop
- One stalk of celery, chop
- 3 cups of chicken broth
- 8 cups of broccoli florets
- 3 tbsp. all-purpose flour
- 2 cups of milk
- ground black pepper to taste

Instructions:

1. Put all the parts together.
2. Two tablespoons of butter should be melted in a bit of stockpot over medium heat. Until tender, cook the onion and celery.
3. For 10 minutes, cover and boil the vegetables and broth.
4. Pour the soup into the mixer's pitcher, filling it more than halfway. Hold the blender's lid down with a folded kitchen towel before turning it on. Before beginning the blender to puree the soup, give it a few quick pulses to move it about.
5. Batch puree until smooth, then transfer to a clean pot. Alternatively, using an immersion mixer, you might purée the broth in the boiling saucepan.
6. In a small saucepan, over low heat, melt the butter 3 Tbsp. Add milk and flour by stirring. Stir until thick and bubbling after adding to broth. Add pepper and then serve.

33.   Old Fashioned Potato Salad

Ingredients:
- Five potatoes
- Three eggs
- 1 cups of chop celery
- ½ cups of chop onion
- ½ cups of sweet pickle relish
- ¼ cups of mayonnaise
- 1 tbsp. prepared mustard
- ¼ tsp. garlic salt
- ¼ tsp. celery salt
- ground black pepper to taste

Instructions:
1. Put all the parts together.
2. Bring to a simmer several cups of salted water in a big pot. Simmer the potatoes for about 15 minutes, or until tender but still firm.
3. Potatoes are peeled, chopped, drained, and chilled.
4. While the potatoes cook, submerge the eggs in a skillet in cold water. Boiling the water, covering it, turning off the heat, and letting the eggs remain in it for 10 to 12 minutes are all acceptable methods.
5. Remove the eggs from the boiling water, let them settle, then peel and chop them.
6. Put the potatoes, eggs, celery, onion, relish, mayo, mustard, relish, garlic, celery, pepper, and pepper in a large bowl and mix well. Combine everything, then put it in the fridge to cool.

34.   Fresh Tomato Soup

Ingredients:

- 4 cups of chop fresh tomatoes
- One slice onion
- Four cloves garlic
- 2 cups of chicken broth
- 2 tbsp. butter
- 2 tbsp. all-purpose flour
- 1 tsp. salt
- 2 tsp. White sugar, or to taste

Instructions:

1. Combine all the components.
2. Tomatoes, a sizable onion, several garlic cloves, and chicken broth should be combined in a stockpot and heated over medium. Cook at a simmer for 20 minutes to allow flavors to meld.
3. After the mixture has been processed in a food processor, remove it from the heat and pour the mixture into a big basin or pan. Any food processor residue ought to be thrown away.
4. In a dry stockpot, melt the butter over low heat. The roux should be stirred in, added, and boiled until it achieves a medium-dark color.
5. To prevent lumps, whisk in a tiny amount gradually. Then, stir in the remaining tomato mixture.
6. Salt and sugar are used to season and taste.

35.   Best Chicken Salad

Ingredients:
- ½ cups of blanched slivered almonds
- ½ cups of mayonnaise
- 1 tbsp. lemon juice
- ¼ tsp. ground black pepper
- 2 cups of chopped, cooked chicken meat
- One stalk of celery, chop

Instructions:
1. Put all the parts together.
2. Add almonds to a skillet for frying. Toast is being shaken constantly over medium-high heat. Keep an eye on them because they burn rapidly.
3. Put the mayonnaise, lemon juice, and pepper in a medium bowl and stir until combined.
4. Combine with chicken, celery, and toasted almonds.

36.   Ukrainian Red Borscht Soup

Ingredients:
- 1 (16 oz.) package of pork sausage
- Three medium beets peeled and shredded
- Three carrots, peeled and shredded
- Three medium baking potatoes, peeled and cubed
- ½ medium head cabbage, cored and shredded
- 1 cups of diced tomatoes, drained
- 1 tbsp. vegetable oil
- One medium onion, chop

- 1 (6 oz.) can of tomato paste
- Eight ¾ cups of water, divided or as needed
- Three cloves garlic, minced
- 1 tsp. white sugar, or to taste
- salt and pepper to taste
- ½ cups of sour cream for topping
- 1 tbsp. Chop fresh parsley for garnish.

Instructions:

1. In a skillet over medium-high heat, crumble pork. Keep stirring until all the red has disappeared. Put the kettle out of its misery and walk away.
2. In a large saucepan, bring 8 cups of water to a boil, covering about half of the contents.
3. Put sausage in the saucepan, cover it, and bring it back to a boil. Beets should be added and cooked until they lose their color. Cook the potatoes and carrots until they are easily pierced with a fork, about 15 minutes.
4. Put the tomato dices and cabbage in the pan.
5. Sauté the onion in the oil until it's soft, about 5 minutes on medium heat. Blend the remaining tomato paste and water, about 3/4 cups. Place in the saucepan.
6. Add the garlic after turning the fire off and covering the broth. Please wait here for five minutes. You can sweeten it with sugar and season it with salt and pepper.
7. Into serving dishes, spoon. Add cilantro and sour cream as a garnish.

37. Homemade Corn Dogs

Ingredients:

- 1 cups of yellow cornmeal
- 1 cups of all-purpose flour
- ¼ cups of white sugar
- Four tsp. baking powder
- ¼ tsp. salt
- ⅛ tsp. black pepper
- 1 cups of milk
- One egg
- 1-quart vegetable oil for frying
- 2 (16 oz.) packages of beef frankfurters
- 16 wooden skewers

Instructions:

1. In a medium basin, combine the cornmeal, flour, sugar, baking powder, salt, and pepper. Stir in the milk and egg to combine.
2. Deep fryer or large saucepan oil to 375 degrees Fahrenheit. 190 °C. Each frankfurter should be stabbed after being dried off with a paper towel in the interim. The batter should thoroughly coat the wieners.
3. Fry two or three corn dogs in hot oil for three minutes until they start to brown. Drain on paper napkins.

38. Broccoli Cheese Soup

Ingredients:

- ½ cups of butter
- One onion, chop
- 1 (16 oz.) package of frozen chop broccoli
- 4 (14.5 oz.) cans of chicken broth
- 1 (1 lb) loaf of processed cheese food, cubed
- 2 cups of milk
- 1 tbsp. garlic powder
- ⅔ cups of cornstarch
- 1 cups of water

Instructions:

1. In a stockpot set over medium heat, melt the butter.
2. When the onion is added, cook it while periodically stirring until soft. Add vegetables and stir. To cook the broccoli, pour in the water and let it simmer for 10 to 15 minutes.
3. Cut cheese into pieces and stir until melted on low heat. Add milk and garlic spice and stir.
4. In a small dish, whisk cornflour and water until thoroughly combined. Add to broth and heat through while frequently stirring until thick.

39. Pasta Salad with Homemade Dressing

Ingredients:

- 1 (8 oz.) package of uncooked tri-color rotini pasta
- 6 oz. pepperoni sausage, diced
- 6 oz. provolone cheese, cubed
- One medium red onion, very thinly sliced and cut into 1-inch pieces
- One small cucumber, thinly sliced
- ¾ cups of chopped green bell pepper
- ¾ cups of chopped red bell pepper
- 1 (6 oz.) can of pitted black olives, drained
- ¼ cups of minced fresh parsley
- ¼ cups of grated Parmesan cheese

Dressing:

- ½ cups of olive oil
- ¼ cups of red wine vinegar
- Two cloves garlic, minced
- 1 tsp. dried basil
- 1 tsp. dried oregano
- ½ tsp. ground mustard seed
- ¼ tsp. Salt
- ⅛ tsp. Ground black pepper

Instructions:

1. Put all the parts together.
2. To prepare, bring a large pot of water to a boil and season it lightly. When the rotini is cooked but still firm to the bite, add

it and simmer for 8 to 10 minutes. Drain again and rinse with cold water.

3. Cooked spaghetti, drained, goes into a large bowl. Including pepperoni, provolone cheese, red onion, cucumber, bell peppers, olives, cilantro, Parmesan cheese, and any other toppings you like is a must.

4. The dressing's components—olive oil, vinegar, garlic, basil, oregano, ground mustard, salt, and pepper—should be combined in a jar with a lid. Shake ferociously while securing the container's cap.

5. Mix the macaroni salad with the dressing after pouring it over it. You can serve it right away, or you can let it chill for up to 8 hours in the fridge.

40. Three Bean Salad

Ingredients:
- 1 (15 oz.) can think of green beans
- 1 lb wax beans
- 1 (15 oz.) can of kidney beans, drained and rinsed
- One onion, sliced into thin rings
- ¾ cups of white sugar, or to taste
- ⅔ cups of distilled white vinegar
- ⅓ cups of vegetable oil
- ½ tsp. salt
- ½ tsp. ground black pepper
- ½ tsp. celery seed

Instructions:
1. Put all the parts together.

2. The following ingredients should be combined: green beans, kidney beans, wax beans, onion, sugar, vinegar, vegetable oil, salt, and celery seed.
3. For at least 12 hours, store in the fridge.

41.   Garlic Bread Spread

Ingredients:
- ½ cups of softened butter
- ¼ cups of grated Parmesan cheese
- Two cloves garlic, minced
- ¼ tsp. dried marjoram
- ¼ tsp. dried basil
- ¼ tsp. fines herbs
- ¼ tsp. dried oregano
- ¼ tsp. dried parsley or to taste
- ground black pepper to taste
- One loaf of unsliced Italian bread

Instructions:
1. After putting the parts together, preheat the oven to 350 °F (175 °C).
2. Butter, Parmesan cheese, basil, marjoram, oregano, parsley, and pepper should all be mixed on a plate.
3. Cut the Italian bread loaf in half lengthwise, then apply the garlic butter mixture on each side. Put these in a roasting pan.
4. Ten to fifteen minutes on the oven's top rack should be enough time for the butter mixture to melt and begin to bubble.

5. Using the broiler in the oven, bake the bread for another one to two minutes, depending on how golden brown you want.

42.   Simple Pasta Salad

Ingredients:

- 1 (16 oz.) package of uncooked rotini pasta
- 1 (16 oz.) bottle of Italian salad dressing
- Two cucumbers chop
- Six tomatoes, chop
- One bunch of green onions, chop
- Four oz. grated Parmesan cheese
- 1 tbsp. Italian seasoning

Instructions:

1. Put all the parts together.
2. To prepare, bring a large pot of water to a boil and season it lightly. Pasta should be cooked for 8-12 minutes in a covered pan until al dente.
3. Combine the cooked pasta, Italian dressing, cucumbers, tomatoes, and green onions in a big dish.
4. Italian spice and Parmesan cheese should be combined in a small dish. The dressing and salad should be combined gently.
5. Cover and chill for at least 30 minutes in the fridge before serving.

43. Hot Dog Mummies

Ingredients:

- Eight hot dogs
- 1 (8 oz.) package of refrigerated crescent
- 1 tsp. Yellow mustard, or as needed

Instructions:

1. Set oven to 350 degrees Fahrenheit. (175 degrees C).
2. The pan containing the hot dogs should be filled with boiling water. Reduce heat to low and simmer for 5 minutes to heat through. Drain.
3. Roll out the crescent dough on a work area and cut it into eight pieces. Each hot dog should have one portion of dough rolled around it to resemble a mummy.
4. Place mustard dots on each for the eyes, nostrils, and mouth. Put hot dogs in a line on a baking pan.
5. Bake in the preheated oven for about 10 minutes, or until the crescent dough is golden brown and flaky.

44. Best Bean Salad

Ingredients:

- 1 (15.5 oz.) can of garbanzo beans, drained
- 1 (14.5 oz.) can of kidney beans, drained
- one (14.5 oz.) can of black beans, drained
- 1 (14.5 oz.) can think of green beans, drained
- 1 (14.5 oz.) can of wax beans, drained
- ½ cups of chopped green pepper
- ½ cups of chop onion

- ½ cups of chop celery
- ¾ cups of white sugar
- ½ cups of salad oil
- ½ cups of vinegar
- ½ tsp. salt
- ½ tsp. Ground black pepper

Instructions:

1. Put all the parts together.
2. To make a hearty meal, mix together a variety of beans (garbanzo, kidney, black, green, wax), vegetables (green pepper, onion, celery), and seasonings.
3. Toss the beans with the sugar, oil, vinegar, salt, and pepper, then drizzle the dressing over the top. Completely combine.
4. Before serving, the salad has to cool for eight to twelve hours.

45. Traditional Gyros

Ingredients:

- One small onion, cut into chunks
- 1 lb ground lamb
- 1 lb ground beef
- 1 tbsp. minced garlic
- 1 tsp. dried oregano
- 1 tsp. ground cumin
- 1 tsp. dried marjoram
- 1 tsp. dried thyme
- 1 tsp. dried rosemary
- 1 tsp. Freshly ground black pepper

- ¼ tsp. sea salt
- 12 tbsp. hummus
- 12 pita bread rounds
- One small head of lettuce, shredded
- One large tomato, sliced
- One large red onion, sliced
- 6 oz. crumbled feta cheese
- 24 tbsp. tzatziki sauce

Instructions:

1. In a food processor, carefully chop the onion. Squeeze the juice from the onion onto a piece of cheesecloth. Add onion to a sizable dish.
2. Using your hands, thoroughly combine the onion, lamb, sirloin, garlic, oregano, cumin, marjoram, thyme, and rosemary. Allow the dish to sit in the fridge, covered in plastic, for at least two hours so the flavors can combine.
3. Set the oven to 325 degrees Fahrenheit. (165 degrees C).
4. The beef mixture should be tacky and finely chopped, so place it in a food processor and process for about a minute. Ensure there are no air pockets when putting the beef mixture into a 7x4-inch loaf pan.
5. Pour enough boiling water around the bread pan to reach halfway up the sides to create a water bath by setting the loaf pan into a roasting pan.
6. Bake in a preheated oven for 45-60 minutes, or until the center is no longer pink. A center reading of at least 165 degrees Fahrenheit on an instant-read thermometer is required. (74 degrees C). Remove any accumulated oil and give it a moment to cool.

7. Slice the prepared gyro meat loaf thinly.

8. Each pita roll should have 1 tbsp. Of hummus on it. Then, to finish off each sandwich, cover it with a few slices of gyro meat, lettuce that has been chopped, tomato and red onion slices, feta cheese crumbles, and two tsp. Of tzatziki sauce.

46. Vermicelli Noodle Bowl

Ingredients:

- ¼ cups of white vinegar
- ¼ cups of fish sauce
- 2 tbsp. white sugar
- 2 tbsp. lime juice
- One clove of garlic, minced
- ¼ tsp. Red pepper flakes
- ½ tsp. canola oil
- 2 tbsp. chop shallots
- Two skewers
- Eight medium shrimp with shells
- 1 (8 oz.) package of rice vermicelli noodles
- one cups of finely chop lettuce
- one cups of bean sprouts
- one English cucumber, cut into 2-inch matchsticks
- ¼ cups of chopped pickled carrots
- ¼ cups of finely chopped daikon radish
- ¼ cups of crushed peanuts
- 3 tbsp. chop cilantro
- 3 tbsp. finely chopped Thai basil
- 3 tbsp. Chop fresh mint

Instructions:

1. Mix the sugar, lime juice, garlic, red pepper flakes, and fish sauce in a small bowl. Throw away the marinade.

2. In a small skillet set over medium heat, warm the oil. When the onions are soft and beginning to caramelize, add them to the pan and stir-fry for about 8 minutes.

3. The grates of a grill should be lightly greased and set to medium heat outside. Each stick should have four shrimp on it, and they should be grilled for one to two minutes on each side or until they turn pink and have a charred exterior. Place away.

4. In a big saucepan, the water is getting hot. Vermicelli noodles should be added once they are flexible and simmered for 12 minutes. Drain and rinse the noodles in cold water while stirring to separate the strands.

5. Each serving dish should have cooked noodles and lettuce, and bean sprouts on one side. A serving of vermicelli will be the end result. Cucumber, carrot, daikon, peanut, cilantro, Thai basil, mint, and caramelized shallots should all be garnished with every meal.

6. Serve with sauce on the side and shrimp skewers. Before serving, pour sauce over the top and thoroughly stir to coat.

47. Curried Egg Sandwiches

Ingredients:

- Four hard-cooked eggs peeled and chopped
- ½ cups of mayonnaise
- 1 tsp. curry powder
- salt and pepper to taste
- Eight slices bread

Instructions:

1. Connect the parts.
2. Mayonnaise and curry powder should be blended in one dish.
3. Slowly incorporate the eggs, and adjust the seasoning with salt and pepper.
4. After dividing evenly between the four pieces, top with the remaining slices of bread.

48. Best Ramen Noodle Salad

Ingredients:

- 2 (3 oz.) Ramen noodles, chicken flavor, packaged in individual servings with seasoning packets set aside.
- ½ cups of raw sunflower seeds
- ½ cups of slivered almonds
- 1 (16 oz.) package of coleslaw mix
- Three green onions, chop

Dressing:

- ½ cups of olive oil
- 3 tbsp. white vinegar

- 1 tbsp. white sugar
- ½ tsp. ground black pepper

Instructions:

1. Set the oven to 350 degrees Fahrenheit. (175 degrees C).
2. Distribute almonds, sunflower seeds, and ramen noodles on a baking tray.
3. Put the noodle mixture on a baking sheet and bake for 10 to 15 minutes, or until the noodles are toasted and fragrant. After cooling it to room temperature, set it away.
4. In a sizable bowl, combine the coleslaw mix and green onions; top with the cooled noodle combination.
5. Produce dressing: In a dish, combine the olive oil, vinegar, sugar, black pepper, and any saved ramen seasoning packets. Mix thoroughly by whisking.
6. Toss the noodle mixture with the dressing so that it is evenly coated.

49.   Zesty Quinoa Salad

Ingredients:

- 2 cups of water
- 1 cups of quinoa
- ¼ cups of extra-virgin olive oil
- Two limes, juiced
- 2 tsp. ground cumin
- 1 tsp. salt
- ½ tsp. red pepper flakes, or more to taste
- 1 ½ cups of halved cherry tomatoes
- one (15 oz.) can of black beans, drained and rinsed

- Five green onions, finely chop
- ¼ cups of chop fresh cilantro
- salt and ground black pepper to taste

Instructions:

1. You must bring water and rice to a boil in a pot. Cover the pan and cook the quinoa on medium-low heat for 10 to 15 minutes or until it is tender and the water has been absorbed. Withhold for chilling.
2. While you wait, prepare a tiny dish with the following ingredients: olive oil, lime juice, cumin, salt, and red pepper flakes.
3. Combine the quinoa, tomatoes, black beans, and green onions on a sizable plate.
4. Mix the dressing with the rice mixture to coat. Add salt and pepper to taste before mixing in the cilantro.
5. Serve immediately or allow the meal to cool in the refrigerator.

50. Easy French Dip Sandwiches

Ingredients:

- Four hoagie rolls split lengthwise
- 1 (10.5 oz.) can of beef consomme
- 1 cups of water
- 1 lb thinly sliced deli roast beef
- 8 slices provolone cheese

Instructions:

1. Three hundred fifty degrees Fahrenheit (175 degrees C) in the oven.
2. Open the sub and spread it out on a baking sheet.
3. In a medium saucepan, bring the water and beef consommé to a boil over medium heat; this will yield a flavorful beef broth.
4. For three minutes, the roast meat is warmed in the broth.
5. Fill the hoagie rolls with meat, and then top with two slices of provolone.
6. Sandwiches with hard cheese can benefit from a brief bake in a hot oven (about five minutes) to soften the cheese.
7. Small cups of heated broth should be provided with sandwiches.

51.   Philly Steak Sandwich

Ingredients:

- ½ tsp. Salt
- ½ tsp. black pepper
- ½ tsp. paprika
- ½ tsp. chili powder
- ½ tsp. onion powder
- ½ tsp. garlic powder
- ½ tsp. dried thyme
- ½ tsp. dried marjoram
- ½ tsp. dried basil
- 1 lb beef sirloin, cut into thin 2-inch strips
- 3 tbsp. vegetable oil

- One onion, sliced
- One green bell pepper, julienned
- 3 oz. Swiss cheese, thinly sliced
- Four hoagie rolls split lengthwise

Instructions:

1. Mix the basil, thyme, marjoram, paprika, onion powder, garlic powder, chili powder, salt, and pepper in a small dish.
2. Put the meat in a very large bowl. Stir to distribute the seasoning mixture on top equally.
3. Put half of the oil in a skillet and heat it over medium heat. Add the cooked beef and continue to sauté. Transfer to a plate.
4. The skillet is heating with the leftover oil. Cook the onions and peppers until soft, then add them to the pan.
5. Set the grill setting on the oven.
6. On the bottoms of 4 rolls, divide the cooked meat. Add onion and green pepper to the layer before adding cheddar slices. On a cookie tray, place.
7. Until the cheese is softened, broil in the preheated oven.
8. Serve the rolls with their top tips.

52.   Caldo de Pollo

Ingredients:

- 5 lbs chicken leg quarters
- 2 gallons water
- 2 tbsp. minced garlic
- 2 tbsp. salt
- 1 tbsp. garlic powder
- 1 cube chicken bouillon
- Four large carrots peeled and cut into large chunks
- Four large potatoes peeled and cut into large chunks
- Four zucchini, sliced into large chunks
- One chayote, cut into large chunks
- One large white onion, cut into large chunks
- ½ bunch of fresh cilantro chop

Instructions:

1. The chicken thighs should be put in a big stockpot with water. Salt, minced garlic, and garlic powder are all added.
2. Cover and simmer rapidly over high heat. Reduce the heat to a boil after cooking for one to two hours.
3. After the poultry bouillon cube has dissolved in the liquid, add the white onion, chayote, carrots, potatoes, and zucchini. Reduce the heat to medium-low, cover the pan, and simmer the potatoes and carrots for 45 to 1 hour.
4. To the broth, add the minced cilantro. For five minutes before serving, simmer.

53. Baked Potato Soup

Ingredients:

- 12 slices bacon
- ⅔ cups of butter or margarine
- ⅔ cups of all-purpose flour
- 7 cups of milk
- Four large baked potatoes, peeled and cubed
- Four green onions, chop
- One ¼ cups of shredded Cheddar cheese
- 1 cups of sour cream
- 1 tsp. salt
- 1 tsp. Ground black pepper

Instructions:

1. Cook the bacon in a large skillet over medium heat until it is evenly browned, about 8 to 10 minutes. On paper towels, pat dry bacon slices; then, crumble and put away.
2. In a Dutch oven or stockpot, melt butter over low heat. Add the flour gradually while whisking to incorporate. Pour milk in slowly while continuously whisking until creamy and thickened.
3. While stirring regularly, add the potatoes and onions and boil. Simmer for 10 minutes at low heat.
4. Add salt, pepper, sour cream, Cheddar cheese, and bacon bits that have been shredded.
5. Cooking and tossing should continue until the cheese melts.

54.   Super-Delicious Zuppa Toscana

Ingredients:

- 1 lb bulk mild Italian sausage
- One ¼ tsp. crushed red pepper flakes
- Four slices of bacon cut into 1/2-inch pieces
- One large onion, diced
- 1 tbsp. minced garlic
- 5 (13.75 oz.) cans of chicken broth
- Six medium potatoes, thinly sliced
- 1 cups of heavy cream
- ¼ bunch fresh spinach, tough stems removed

Instructions:

1. Italian sausage and red pepper flakes should be cooked in a Dutch oven for 10 to 15 minutes or until the meat is crumbly, browned, and no longer pink. Drain, and then separate.
2. In the same Dutch oven, the pork has to cook for 10 minutes at medium heat. Place the bacon and a few tablespoons of the drippings in the bottom of the Dutch oven after they have been drained.
3. Stir in the garlic and onions. The onions should be tender and transparent after five minutes of cooking.
4. Before adding the chicken stock, stir and bring to a boil. The potatoes should be boiled for 20 minutes, or until fork-tender. After reducing the heat to medium, add the cream along with the cooked beef and spinach and stir.
5. Beef and spinach should be heated thoroughly after being cooked and stirred.

55.   Reuben Sandwich

Ingredients:

- Eight slices of rye bread
- ½ cups of Thousand Island dressing
- Eight pieces of Swiss cheese
- Eight slices deli sliced corned beef
- 1 cups of sauerkraut, drained
- 2 tbsp. butter softened

Instructions:

1. Preheat a big skillet or pan over medium heat.
2. Spread the Thousand Island dressing on the underside of the bread slices. Four pieces of bread should be topped with one slice of Swiss cheese, two cuts of corned meat, one-fourth cups of sauerkraut, and a second slice of Swiss cheese. Spread the remaining dressing on the bread slices. Spread butter on the outside of the bread.
3. Put the buttered side down of each sandwich on the hot grill and spread the butter on top. If you want golden brown grill marks on both sides, it takes about 5 minutes per side. Serve hot

56. Pasta Salad

Ingredients:

- 1 lb tri-colored spiral pasta
- 1 (16 oz.) bottle of Italian-style salad dressing
- 6 tbsp. salad seasoning mix
- 2 cups of cherry tomatoes, diced
- One green bell pepper, chop
- One red bell pepper, diced
- ½ yellow bell pepper, chop
- 1 (2.25 oz.) can of black olives, chop

Instructions:

1. Assemble all the components.
2. A large pot of mildly salted water should be brought to a boil. Pasta should be cooked in boiling water for 10 to 12 minutes, stirring periodically, until tender to the bite but firm. Drain, then rinse under cold water.
3. Italian dressing and salad seasoning blend should be thoroughly combined in a bowl. Combine the pasta, tomatoes, bell peppers, and olives in a salad dish.
4. Sprinkle lettuce with dressing, then toss to combine.
5. Salad should be chilled for eight to twelve hours.

57. Sloppy Joes

Ingredients:

- 1 lb lean ground beef
- ¼ cups of chop onion
- ¼ cups of chopped green bell pepper
- ¾ cups of ketchup, or to taste
- 1 tbsp. brown sugar, or to taste
- 1 tsp. yellow mustard, or to taste
- ½ tsp. garlic powder
- salt and ground black pepper to taste
- Six hamburger buns, split

Instructions:

1. Heat a huge skillet to a medium temperature. Brown ground beef until some oil begins to render, about 3 to 4 minutes in a hot skillet with occasional stirring. Add the onion and bell pepper once the meat is done cooking and continue simmering for another 3–5 minutes, or until the vegetables are tender.
2. After seasoning with salt and pepper, stir in the ketchup, brown sugar, mustard, and garlic powder. For 20–30 minutes at a medium simmer.
3. Give each bun an equal amount of the beef mixture.

58.   Taco Bell Seasoning Copycat

Ingredients:

- 1 tbsp. dried onion flakes
- 1 tsp. all-purpose flour
- 1 tsp. beef bouillon granules
- 1 tsp. garlic salt
- 1 tsp. ground cumin
- 1 tsp. paprika
- 1 tsp. chili powder
- ¼ tsp. cayenne pepper
- ¼ tsp. white sugar

Instructions:

1. Combine sugar, cumin, paprika, chili powder, cayenne pepper, garlic salt, onion flakes, flour, and bouillon granules in a dish.

59.   Slow Cooker Buffalo Chicken Sandwiches

Ingredients:

- Four skinless, boneless chicken breast halves
- 1 (17.5 fluid oz.) bottle of Buffalo wing sauce divided
- ½ (1 oz.) package of dry ranch salad dressing mix
- 2 tbsp. butter
- Six hoagie rolls split lengthwise

Instructions:

1. Add the chicken breasts, 3/4 of the wing sauce, and ranch dressing mixture in the slow cooker.
2. Cook on Low for six to seven hours with the cover on.
3. Utilizing two forks, shred poultry in the cooker. Add butter and stir.
4. Hoagie rolls should be topped with sauce and shredded poultry. Serve alongside any leftover Buffalo sauce.

Chapter 3:- Dinner Recipe

60.   Spaghetti Bolognese

Ingredients:

- 1 lb ground beef
- One onion, diced
- Two cloves garlic, minced
- One can of crushed tomatoes (28 oz)
- One can of tomato sauce (15 oz)
- 2 tbsp. tomato paste
- 1 tsp. dried basil
- 1 tsp. dried oregano
- 1/2 tsp. salt
- 1/4 tsp. black pepper
- 1 lb spaghetti
- Parmesan cheese, grated

Directions:

1. The ground beef should be cooked until browned, stirring periodically, in a big skillet over medium heat. Get rid of any extra weight.
2. Add the onion to the skillet, beef, and minced garlic when translucent.
3. The pan should now contain crushed tomatoes, tomato sauce, paste, basil, oregano, salt, and black pepper. To blend, stir.
4. Simmer the sauce for 20 to 30 minutes, whisking now and then.
5. The pasta should be prepared as directed on the packaging. Spaghetti that has been drained should be added to the sauce in the pan. Combine by tossing.
6. If preferred, top the spaghetti with freshly grated Parmesan cheese.

61.   Lemon Garlic Chicken

Ingredients:

- Four boneless, skinless chicken breasts
- Salt and pepper, to taste
- 2 tbsp. olive oil
- 2 tbsp. butter
- Four cloves garlic, minced
- 1/4 cups of chicken broth
- Juice of 1 lemon
- Lemon slices, for garnish
- Fresh parsley, chop, for garnish

Directions:

1. Salt and pepper both sides of the chicken breasts.
2. In a large pan over medium heat, olive oil should be warmed. After cooking the chicken breasts in the pan for 5 to 6 minutes on each side, they must be thoroughly cooked and golden brown.
3. After cooking, transfer the chicken to a serving platter.
4. Butter should be melted in the same skillet over medium heat. Cook the garlic in the skillet for 1-2 minutes, stirring frequently.
5. Put the garlic in a skillet and add the chicken stock and lemon juice. Simmer the concoction for 2–3 minutes, or until it thickens.
6. Re-add the chicken to the sauce-filled pan and cover it with sauce.
7. The fowl should be garnished with lemon slices and fresh parsley.

62.   Grilled Steak with Chimichurri Sauce

Ingredients:

- 2-3 lbs. flank steak
- Salt and pepper, to taste
- 1/4 cups of olive oil
- 1/4 cups of red wine vinegar
- 1/2 cups of fresh parsley leaves
- 1/4 cups of fresh cilantro leaves
- Four garlic cloves
- One shallot, chop

- 1/4 tsp. red pepper flakes
- 1/2 tsp. ground cumin

Directions:

1. On both sides, season the flank sirloin with salt and pepper.
2. Heat the grill to a high temperature.
3. In a blender or food processor, combine the olive oil, red wine vinegar, herbs, garlic, shallot, pepper flakes, and cumin. Pulse to thoroughly mix the components.
4. Grill the steak for 4-5 minutes on each side or until it is done to your liking.
5. After removing the sirloin from the grill, rest for five to ten minutes.
6. Serve the sirloin with the chimichurri sauce after cutting it against the grain.

63.   Vegetable Stir-Fry

Ingredients:

- 2 tbsp. vegetable oil
- One red bell pepper, sliced
- One green bell pepper, sliced
- One yellow onion, sliced
- Two carrots, sliced
- One broccoli crown, chop
- 1 tbsp. soy sauce
- 1 tbsp. oyster sauce
- 1 tsp. sesame oil
- 1 tsp. cornstarch
- Salt and pepper, to taste

Directions:

1. In a large skillet or wok, heat the vegetable oil over high heat.
2. For two to three minutes, or until they soften, stir-fry the sliced bell peppers and onion in the pan.
3. Stir-fry the chopped broccoli and thinly sliced carrots for two to three minutes.
4. Mix the cornstarch, soy sauce, oyster sauce, sesame oil, salt, and pepper on a small plate.
5. After the sauce has reduced and the vegetables are coated, remove the pan from the heat and serve.
6. If you'd like, serve the stir-fried vegetables with rice or noodles.

64.   Baked Salmon with Lemon and Herbs

Ingredients:

- Four salmon fillets (6 oz each)
- Salt and pepper, to taste
- 2 tbsp. olive oil
- 2 tbsp. chop fresh parsley
- 1 tbsp. chop fresh dill
- One lemon, sliced

Directions:

1. Set the oven to 400°F.
2. On both sides, season the salmon pieces with salt and pepper.
3. Salmon fillets should be placed skin-side down in a baking tray.
4. Olive oil should be drizzled over the salmon pieces before adding parsley and dill.

5. Overlay the salmon fillets with the lemon segments.
6. Bake the salmon for 12–15 minutes, or until it is easily flaked with a fork.
7. If preferred, serve the baked salmon with more lemon slices.

65.   Chicken Fajitas

Ingredients:
- One lb. boneless, skinless chicken breasts, sliced
- Salt and pepper, to taste
- 2 tbsp. vegetable oil
- One red bell pepper, sliced
- One green bell pepper, sliced
- One yellow onion, sliced
- 1 tbsp. chili powder
- 1 tsp. ground cumin
- 1/2 tsp. garlic powder
- 1/2 tsp. paprika
- 1/4 tsp. cayenne pepper
- Flour tortillas
- Shredded cheese
- Sour cream
- Salsa

Directions:
1. Salt and pepper the chicken breast slices as desired.
2. To prepare the vegetable oil, heat a large pan over medium heat.
3. After 6 to 8 minutes, add the chicken slices to the pan and finish cooking them.

4. The chicken should be removed from the skillet and stored.
5. Slices of bell pepper and onion can be added to the same pan. After three to four minutes of cooking, they ought to be tender.
6. Toss in some heat with some chili powder, garlic powder, paprika, and cayenne pepper. Stir the mixture.
7. Add the vegetables and poultry to the skillet while stirring.
8. Warm flour tortillas, salsa, sour cream, and shredded cheese should be served with the chicken fajita filling.

66.   One-Pot Beef Stew

Ingredients:

- 2 lbs beef stew meat, cubed
- Salt and pepper, to taste
- 2 tbsp. olive oil
- One onion, chop
- Four garlic cloves minced
- 2 cups of beef broth
- 2 cups of water
- Two carrots peeled and chopped
- Two celery stalks, chop
- Two potatoes peeled and chopped
- 1 tbsp. tomato paste
- 1 tsp. dried thyme
- One bay leaf

Directions:

1. Salt and pepper the flesh for the beef stew.

2. In a large skillet or Dutch oven, heat the olive oil over medium heat.
3. The beef stew flesh should be added to the pool and cooked for about 5 minutes or until browned on all sides.
4. Add the chopped onion and garlic to the saucepan and cook for two to three minutes, or until the onion is soft and the garlic is fragrant.
5. Stirring is required after adding the water and meat broth.
6. Add the tomato paste, dried thyme, and bay leaf to the saucepan and the diced potatoes, carrots, and celery.
7. Turn the heat down to medium and cover the pot to let the stew simmer for a while.
8. The beef and veggies should be tender after simmering the stew for about an hour or two.
9. Before serving, take the bay leaf out.

67.   Creamy Tomato Soup with Grilled Cheese Sandwiches

Ingredients:
For the soup:

- 1 tbsp. olive oil
- One onion, chop
- Two garlic cloves minced
- Two cans (28 oz each) of crushed tomatoes
- 2 cups of chicken broth
- 1/2 cups of heavy cream
- Salt and pepper, to taste

For the grilled cheese sandwiches:

- Eight slices bread
- Four slices of cheddar cheese
- Butter, for spreading on the bread

Directions:

1. The olive oil should be heated over medium flame in a big saucepan or Dutch oven.
2. Add the chopped onion and garlic to the saucepan and cook for two to three minutes, or until the onion is soft and the garlic is fragrant.
3. Crushed tomatoes and chicken stock should be added, and they should be combined.
4. The broth should simmer for 15 to 20 minutes.
5. The soup should be pureed until smooth using an immersion mixer or by transferring it in batches to a blender.
6. Salt and pepper to taste, then stir in the heavy cream.
7. Heat a pan to medium heat to prepare the grilled cheese sandwiches.
8. Spread butter on only one side of each slice of bread.
9. Place a slice of cheese between two pieces of bread with the buttered sides facing out.
10. When the cheese has melted and the bread is golden brown, cook the sandwiches in the pan for two to three minutes on each side.
11. Grilled cheese sandwiches should be presented with rich tomato sauce.

68. Tacos al Pastor

Ingredients:

- 2 lbs boneless pork shoulder, sliced into thin strips
- 1/2 cups of pineapple juice
- 1/4 cups of orange juice
- 1/4 cups of lime juice
- 1/4 cups of white vinegar
- 1/4 cups of achiote paste
- 1 tbsp. dried oregano
- 1 tbsp. ground cumin
- 1 tbsp. chili powder
- 1 tsp. salt
- 1/2 tsp. black pepper
- One onion, chop
- Two cloves garlic, minced
- 2 tbsp. vegetable oil
- 1/2 cups of chop fresh cilantro
- 12-16 small corn tortillas
- Pineapple chunks and chopped onion for serving

Directions:

1. In a large bowl should blend the pineapple, orange, lime, white vinegar, achiote paste, dried oregano, ground cumin, chili powder, salt, and black pepper. By whisking, completely combine.
2. The sauce has to be applied and coated with the sliced pork shoulder. Place the dish in the refrigerator overnight, covering it with plastic wrap for at least two hours.
3. High heat should be applied to a skillet or grill pan.

4. Vegetable oil should be heated over medium heat in a large skillet.
5. When you're ready, throw in some onions and garlic and let them sweat for a few minutes.
6. Cook the pork for 5–7 minutes, until browned and cooked through, stirring occasionally.
7. Pork, chopped fresh cilantro, pineapple segments, onion, and warm tortillas.

69. Mississippi Chicken

Ingredients:
- 2 lbs skinless, boneless chicken breasts
- 1 (1 oz.) ranch dressing mix in a packet (like Hidden Valley Ranch®)
- 1 (16 oz.) jar of sliced pepperoncini peppers, drained
- 4 tbsp. Unsalted butter, sliced

Instructions:
1. The oven temperature is set to 350 degrees Fahrenheit. (175 degrees C).
2. The poultry should be placed in the bottom of a big Dutch oven and seasoned with ranch seasoning mix. Spread butter, pepperoncini peppers, and 1/2 cups of pepper juice over the chicken. The chicken should be fork tender within an hour and a half and undercover in a preheated oven. The internal temperature should read 165 degrees Fahrenheit on an instant-read thermometer. (74 degrees C).
3. Five minutes should pass. Shred the chicken using two forks.

70. Stout-Braised Lamb Shanks

Ingredients:

- 1 tbsp. vegetable oil
- Four lamb shanks
- One onion, chop
- Four cloves of garlic, chop
- Two carrots, chop
- Two celery ribs, chop
- 2 tbsp. tomato paste
- 1 (14 oz.) can of beef broth
- 1 (12 fluid oz.) bottle of stout or porter
- Three sprigs of fresh thyme
- Three sprigs of fresh parsley
- One bay leaf
- One sprig of fresh rosemary
- Salt and pepper to taste

Instructions:

1. Oil should be heated in a Dutch oven or other large, wide pot until it smokes over medium-high heat. Lamb shanks should be browned on all sides in hot oil for about ten minutes. Lamb shanks should be taken out and set aside. Get rid of extra oil.

2. Add onion and garlic to the Dutch oven and heat over medium heat. An onion that has been softened and made transparent should have taken about 5 minutes to fry and stir. After adding tomato puree, carrots, and celery, cook for five more minutes.

3. Put the lamb shanks in a Dutch oven and add the beer and stock. Bind a bundle of thyme, parsley, and bay leaf with

kitchen twine before adding it to lamb shanks and bringing it to a simmer.

4. Stirring occasionally, lower the heat to medium-low, cover the pan, and simmer the lamb for two to three hours. Season with salt and pepper, and add the rosemary leaves during the last 10 minutes of cooking. Remove the rosemary plant bundle and sprig before serving.

71. Corned Beef Roast

Ingredients:
- 1 (5 1/2 lb) corned beef brisket with spice packet
- Seven small potatoes, peeled and diced
- Four carrots, peeled and diced
- One medium onion, diced
- Three cloves garlic, chop

Instructions:
1. The oven temperature is set to 300 degrees Fahrenheit. (150 degrees C).
2. The corned beef brisket should be placed in the middle of a roasting pan. Onions and garlic should be sprinkled on top of the meat, surrounded by potatoes and carrots. Sprinkle the seasoning packet's contents over the meat after adding water to almost submerge the potatoes. Cover with a lid or a substantial metal sheet.
3. Corned beef must roast in a preheated oven for 5 to 6 hours or until a blade can easily pierce it.

72. Lasagna Flatbread

Ingredients:

- 1 (15 oz.) container of ricotta cheese
- 1 (8 oz.) package of shredded mozzarella cheese divided
- 1 (3 oz.) package of Parmesan cheese
- One egg
- 2 tsp. Italian seasoning
- 1 lb sausage
- ½ (26 oz.) jar marinara sauce
- Six flatbreads

Instructions:

1. The oven should be set to 375 degrees. (190 degrees C).
2. Combine the egg, ricotta cheese, half of the mozzarella cheese, Parmesan cheese, and Italian spice in a dish.
3. Cooking sausage in a skillet on medium heat for 5 to 10 minutes, or until no longer pink, is recommended. Drain. Mix in the tomato puree.
4. Place a sixth of the cheese mixture evenly across each flatbread, followed by the meat mixture. On top, sprinkle the remaining mozzarella cheese.
5. Bake in a preheated oven for 10 to 15 minutes or until the cheese is melted and melted.

73.   Basic Air Fryer Hot Dogs

Ingredients:

- Four hot dog buns
- Four hot dogs

Instructions:

1. Obtain an air burner temperature of 400°F. 200 °C.
2. Place the buns in the air fryer basket in a single layer. The buns should be cooked for about 2 minutes or until crisp. The buns are placed on a dish.
3. Cook the hot dogs for 3 minutes in a single layer in the air fryer basket. Hot dogs and warm bread are served.

74.   Homemade Mac and Cheese

Ingredients:
Macaroni and Cheese:

- Eight oz. uncooked elbow macaroni
- ¼ cups of salted butter
- 3 tbsp. all-purpose flour
- 2 ½ cups of milk, or more as needed
- 2 cups of shredded sharp Cheddar cheese
- ½ cups of finely grated Parmesan cheese
- Salt and ground black pepper to taste

Bread Crumb Topping:

- 2 tbsp. salted butter
- ½ cups of dry bread crumbs

- One pinch of ground paprika

Instructions:

1. The preheated oven's temperature should be 350 degrees. temperature of 175 C. Prepare a greased 8-by-8-inch baking dish.

2. Preparing mac and cheese: Bring several large, lightly salted water containers to a boil. The spaghetti will keep cooking in the oven. When the macaroni is fork-tender but still firm, add it to the pot and boil for about 8 minutes, stirring regularly. Drain, then place on the baking sheet.

3. In a medium skillet, melt a quarter cup of butter over low heat while the spaghetti cooks. Once the flour has been added, whisk the mixture for 3 to 5 minutes or until it resembles paste and turns golden.

4. Before simmering, 2 1/2 cups of milk should be gradually incorporated into the flour mixture. Add the finely grated Parmesan and Cheddar cheeses and salt and pepper. Melt the cheese and thicken the sauce by cooking the mixture for 3 to 5 minutes while stirring it occasionally. Extra milk of up to a half cup may be added if needed. Cheese sauce and pasta must be properly mixed.

5. Two tablespoons of butter should be melted over medium heat in a skillet before the bread crumbs are added. Cooking and stirring the bread crumbs until they are coated and toasted evenly is required. After scattering bread crumbs over the macaroni and cheese, sprinkle paprika over it.

6. The coating should be golden brown, and the macaroni and cheese should be bubbling after 30 minutes of baking.

75. Slow Cooker Texas Pulled Pork

Ingredients:

- 1 tsp. vegetable oil
- 1 (4 lb) pork shoulder roast
- 1 cups of barbeque sauce
- ½ cups of apple cider vinegar
- ½ cups of chicken broth
- ¼ cups of light brown sugar
- 1 tbsp. prepared yellow mustard
- 1 tbsp. Worcestershire sauce
- 1 tbsp. chili powder
- One extra large onion, chop
- Two large cloves of garlic, crushed
- 1 ½ tsp. dried thyme
- Eight hamburger buns, split
- 2 tbsp. Butter, or as needed

Instructions:

1. In the bottom of the slow cooker, add some vegetable oil. Put the vinegar, BBQ sauce, and chicken stock in the slow cooker with the pork roast. Add the mustard, thyme, onion, garlic, Worcestershire sauce, chili pepper, brown sugar, and yellow to the mixture. The pork should easily fall apart when tested with a skewer after cooking for 10-12 hours on Low or 5-6 hours on High.

2. After taking the pork out of the slow cooker, use two forks to shred the meat. The shredded pork can be tossed with the juices and placed in the slow cooker.

3. Both beef bread halves should be brushed with butter. Toast the bread and butter in a skillet over medium heat until browned. Insert buttered bread containing pulled pork.

76. Slow Cooker Beef Stew

Ingredients:

- Two lbs of beef stew meat cut into 1-inch pieces
- ¼ cups of all-purpose flour
- ½ tsp. salt
- ½ tsp. ground black pepper
- 1 ½ cups of beef broth
- Four medium carrots, sliced
- Three medium potatoes, diced
- One medium onion, chop
- One stalk of celery, chop
- 1 tsp. Worcestershire sauce
- 1 tsp. ground paprika
- One clove of garlic, minced
- One large bay leaf

Instructions:

1. To the slow cooker, add the beef.
2. Mix the flour, salt, and pepper in a separate bowl. After adding the sauce to the beef, stir it.
3. Stir in the meat broth with the celery, carrots, potatoes, onions, bay leaf, Worcestershire sauce, and paprika.
4. Simmer the meat covered on low for 8-12 hours, or on high for 4-6 hours, until it is fork-tender.

77.   Chicken Caesar Salad

Ingredients:
For the salad:

- Four chicken breasts
- Salt and pepper, to taste
- 2 tbsp. olive oil
- 8 cups of chop romaine lettuce
- 1 cups of croutons
- 1/2 cups of grated Parmesan cheese

For the dressing:

- 1/2 cups of mayonnaise
- 2 tbsp. Dijon mustard
- 2 tbsp. lemon juice
- 1 tbsp. Worcestershire sauce
- Two garlic cloves minced
- 1/4 cups of grated Parmesan cheese
- Salt and pepper, to taste

Directions:
1. The oven should be set at 375°F.
2. Chicken breasts need seasoning with salt and pepper.
3. Melt the olive oil in a big oven-safe pan over medium-high heat.
4. Cooking time for the chicken breasts in the skillet should be two to three minutes per side or until browned.
5. Chicken can be baked for 20–25 minutes in the oven, depending on how done you like it.

6. After removing the fowl from the skillet should, rest for five minutes.
7. Combine the mayonnaise, Dijon mustard, lemon juice, Worcestershire sauce, minced garlic, grated Parmesan cheese, salt, and pepper in a small dish.
8. Thin chunks of chicken breasts should be cut from them.
9. Mix chopped romaine lettuce, croutons, and grated Parmesan cheese in a big bowl.
10. Toss the lettuce with the dressing and serve..
11. Slices of chicken breast should be garnished on top of the salad.

78. Shrimp Scampi

Ingredients:

- 1 lb linguine
- 4 tbsp. unsalted butter
- 4 tbsp. olive oil
- Four garlic cloves minced
- 1/2 tsp. red pepper flakes
- 1 lb large shrimp, peeled and deveined
- 1/2 cups of dry white wine
- 1/4 cups of freshly squeezed lemon juice
- 1/4 cups of chopped fresh parsley
- Salt and pepper, to taste

Directions:

1. Follow the instructions on the linguine box for cooking. Separate and drain.

2. Butter should be melted in a large pan over low to medium heat.
3. For 1-2 minutes, or until fragrant, heat the olive oil in a skillet and add the garlic and red pepper flakes.
4. After 2–3 minutes, the shrimp should turn pink and be fully cooked in the pan.
5. The shrimp should be removed from the pan and set aside.
6. Bring the white wine and lemon juice to a boil in the pan.
7. Reduce heat and simmer for 5–7 minutes, or until sauce thickens.
8. Toss the cooked linguine and shrimp in the sauce in the pan after adding them.
9. Add the parsley that has been minced and season with salt and pepper to taste.
10. Quickly serve.

79.   Spicy Sausage and Vegetable Skillet

Ingredients:
- 1 lb spicy Italian sausage, sliced
- One red bell pepper, sliced
- One green bell pepper, sliced
- One yellow onion, sliced
- Two zucchini sliced
- Two garlic cloves minced
- 1/2 tsp. dried oregano
- 1/2 tsp. dried basil
- 1/2 tsp. dried thyme
- Salt and pepper, to taste

- 2 tbsp. olive oil
- 1/4 cups of chopped fresh parsley

Directions:

1. Warm the olive oil in a large skillet over medium heat.
2. Sliced sausage should be added to the pan and cooked for three to four minutes or until browned.
3. Sausage should be taken out of the skillet and put away.
4. Salt, pepper, oregano, basil, thyme, onion, bell peppers, zucchini, and garlic can all be added to the pan.
5. For 6-8 minutes, or until vegetables are tender.
6. Put the cooked meat back in the pan and mix it with the sauce.
7. Serve hot and top with cilantro that has been chopped.

80.   Eggplant Parmesan

Ingredients:

- Two large eggplants, sliced into 1/2-inch rounds
- 2 cups of breadcrumbs
- 1/2 cups of grated parmesan cheese
- Two eggs, beaten
- 2 cups of marinara sauce
- 1 lb fresh mozzarella, sliced
- Salt and pepper, to taste
- 1/4 cups of chopped fresh basil

Directions:

1. The oven should be set at 375°F.
2. Parchment paper should be used to line a baking sheet.

3. Combine the breadcrumbs and parmesan in a separate bowl.

4. The beaten eggs should be applied to each eggplant slice first, then the breadcrumb mixture.

5. Place the eggplant slices on the baking sheet that has been prepared.

6. If you want the eggplant to be crispy and golden brown, bake it for 15–20 minutes.

7. Spread some marinara sauce on the bottom of a 9x13 baking dish.

8. After the eggplant is done baking, top the dish with the mozzarella slices.

9. Once all of the eggplant pieces have been used, keep piling them.

10. On top, spread a final layer of mozzarella cheese and marinara sauce.

11. Wait 20-25 minutes in the oven for the cheese to melt and bubble.

12. Serve hot, and sprinkle chopped fresh basil over top.

81.   Beef and Broccoli Stir-Fry

Ingredients:
- 1 lb flank steak, thinly sliced
- 1 lb broccoli florets
- 3 tbsp. vegetable oil
- Three garlic cloves minced
- 1 tbsp. grated fresh ginger
- 1/2 cups of beef broth
- 1/4 cups of soy sauce

- 2 tbsp. cornstarch
- 2 tbsp. water
- Salt and pepper, to taste
- Cooked rice for serving

Directions:
1. Two tsp. of the vegetable oil should be heated to a high temperature in a sizable skillet or wok.
2. Add the sliced flank beef to the pan and cook for another two to three minutes, or until browned.
3. It's time to stop cooking the steak and put it away.
4. The skillet should now contain the final tbsp. of vegetable oil.
5. Cook the garlic and ginger for another minute or two until fragrant.
6. Once the broccoli florets have reached the desired tender-crispness, add them to the pan.
7. Put the beef stock, soy sauce, cornstarch, and water into a small bowl.
8. When the sauce has boiled, pour it into the pan.
9. Reduce heat and simmer sauce for 2-3 minutes, or until desired thickness is reached.
10. Toss the cooked flank beef with the sauce in the pan.
11. Pepper and salt the dish to your liking.
12. Spread hot rice on top.

82.   Stuffed Peppers

Ingredients:

- Four bell peppers, any color
- 1 lb ground beef
- One onion, chop
- Two cloves garlic, minced
- 1 cups of cooked rice
- 1 cups of tomato sauce
- 1 tsp. dried basil
- 1 tsp. dried oregano
- Salt and pepper, to taste
- 1 cups of shredded cheddar cheese

Directions:

1. The oven should be set at 375°F.
2. Cut off the stems and bottoms of the peppers, then remove and discard the stems, seeds, and membranes.
3. Brown the ground beef in a large skillet over medium heat.
4. Minced garlic and sliced onion should be cooked for 5 minutes in a skillet until soft.
5. Add the tomato sauce, salt, pepper, dried basil, dried oregano, and prepared rice.
6. The meat and rice
7. The combination should be put inside the bell peppers.
8. The filled peppers should be placed in a baking dish and covered with foil.
9. The peppers should be baked for 30-35 minutes or until tender.

10. Take the peppers out of the paper and top them with some grated cheddar cheese.
11. Re-bake the peppers in the oven for 5 to 10 minutes after the cheese has dissolved and started to bubble.
12. Serve hot.

83.   Ratatouille

Ingredients:
- One onion, chop
- Two cloves garlic, minced
- 2 tbsp. olive oil
- One eggplant, diced
- One zucchini, diced
- One yellow squash, diced
- One red bell pepper, diced
- One yellow bell pepper, diced
- One can (14 oz) diced tomatoes
- 1 tbsp. tomato paste
- 1 tsp. dried basil
- 1 tsp. dried oregano
- Salt and pepper, to taste

Directions:
1. 375°F should be the oven's temperature.
2. Olive oil, in a large skillet, should be heated over medium heat.
3. The onion and garlic should be cooked through after 5 minutes in the pan.

4. The cooking time for the red, yellow, and other veggies will depend on how tender you like your vegetables. Cook the vegetables for 10 to 12 minutes after adding them to the pan.
5. In a bowl, mix the chopped tomatoes with the dried herbs (the oregano, basil, salt, and pepper).
6. The components should be arranged on a sizable baking sheet.
7. Bake the dish, covered with foil, for 30-35 minutes or until the veggies are thoroughly cooked and soft.
8. Heated food.

84.   Chicken Tikka Masala

Ingredients:
For the chicken:

- Two lbs boneless, skinless chicken breasts cut into bite-sized pieces
- 1/2 cups of plain yogurt
- 2 tbsp. lemon juice
- 1 tbsp. ground cumin
- 1 tbsp. ground coriander
- 1 tbsp. garam masala
- 1 tsp. turmeric
- 1/2 tsp. cayenne pepper
- Salt and pepper, to taste

For the sauce:

- 2 tbsp. vegetable oil
- One onion, chop

- Two cloves garlic, minced
- 2 tsp. grated fresh ginger
- 1 tbsp. garam masala
- 1 tsp. paprika
- 1/2 tsp. ground cinnamon
- 1/2 tsp. ground turmeric
- One can (14 oz) crushed tomatoes
- 1 cups of heavy cream
- Salt and pepper, to taste
- Cooked rice for serving

Directions:

1. Combine the yogurt, lemon juice, garam masala, cumin, coriander, turmeric, cayenne pepper, salt, and pepper in a large saucepan.
2. After adding the poultry pieces to the bowl, stir the marinade together.
3. Put the lid on the jar and chill it for at least an hour, preferably overnight.
4. Four hundred degrees Fahrenheit should be set for the oven.
5. Place the pieces of marinated chicken on a baking sheet.
6. 20 to 25 minutes should be enough time to roast the whole chicken.
7. Warm the oil for cooking in a large skillet over low to medium heat.
8. The chop onion should be tender after five minutes of cooking.
9. Minced garlic and newly grated ginger should be combined in the skillet. Cook until aromatic, about 1-2 minutes.

10. To the pan, add the garam masala, paprika, cinnamon, and turmeric powders.
11. Cook until aromatic, about 1-2 minutes.
12. After that, incorporate rich milk and chop tomatoes.
13. Season the marinade with salt and pepper to taste.
14. The sauce should thicken after ten to fifteen minutes of simmering.
15. After the chicken has baked, toss it with the sauce in the pan.
16. Serve with hot rice.

85. Grilled Teriyaki Chicken Skewers

Ingredients:
- One lb boneless, skinless chicken breasts cut into cubes
- 1/2 cups of teriyaki sauce
- 1/4 cups of honey
- 2 tbsp. rice vinegar
- 1 tbsp. sesame oil
- Salt and pepper, to taste

Directions:
1. In a big dish, combine the teriyaki sauce, honey, rice vinegar, sesame oil, salt, and pepper.
2. Throw the chicken into the marinade and toss to coat.
3. Cover the container and refrigerate it for at least an hour and up to a full day.
4. Marinated chicken is skewered and used.
5. After 8 to 10 minutes on the grill over medium-high heat, the chicken kebabs ought to be thoroughly cooked.

6. Rice and your preferred vegetables, served hot.

86. Black Bean and Corn Quesadillas

Ingredients:
- Four large flour tortillas
- One can (15 oz) of black beans, drained and rinsed
- 1 cups of frozen corn kernels
- 1/2 cups of chop fresh cilantro
- 1/4 tsp. ground cumin
- 1/4 tsp. chili powder
- Salt and pepper, to taste
- 1 cups of shredded cheddar cheese
- Sour cream for serving

Directions:
1. Combine the black beans, corn, chop cilantro, ground cumin, chili powder, salt, and pepper in a sizable dish.
2. A giant skillet should be heated to medium.
3. One tortilla should be placed in the pan with half the shredded cheddar cheese on top.
4. Over the cheese, spoon half of the black bean and corn combination.
5. Add a second tortilla and gently push it down with a spatula.
6. Quesadillas need to be cooked for two to three minutes per side, or until the cheese has melted and the bread is crisp.
7. Make a second quesadilla by repeating the process with the leftover ingredients.
8. Serve the quesadillas hot with sour cream after cutting them into pieces.

87. Beef and Mushroom Stroganoff

Ingredients:

- One lb beef sirloin, cut into thin strips
- 1 tbsp. vegetable oil
- One onion, finely chop
- 8 oz sliced mushrooms
- Two cloves garlic, minced
- 1 tbsp. tomato paste
- 1 cups of beef broth
- 1/2 cups of sour cream
- Salt and pepper, to taste
- Cooked egg noodles for serving

Directions:

1. Vegetable oil should be heated to a medium-high temperature in a sizable pan.
2. The beef pieces should be added to the skillet until well browned.
3. It's time to stop cooking the beef and put the skillet away.
4. For about 5 minutes, or until soft, sauté the chopped onion in the pan.
5. After adding the mushrooms and garlic, let them cook for 5 minutes.
6. Add the meat broth and tomato paste after mixing.
7. Simmer the liquid for 10–15 minutes, or until it reaches the desired thickness.
8. Add the sour cream after seasoning to taste with salt and pepper.
9. Heat the meat once more in the skillet.

10. With steaming egg noodles, serve.

88. Baked Ziti with Sausage and Ricotta

Ingredients:
- 1 lb ziti pasta
- 1 lb sweet Italian sausage, casings removed
- One jar (24 oz) of marinara sauce
- 1 cups of ricotta cheese
- 1 cups of shredded mozzarella cheese
- 1/2 cups of grated Parmesan cheese
- Salt and pepper, to taste
- Chop fresh basil for serving

Directions:
1. Turn the oven on to 375°F.
2. Cook ziti according to package directions until al dente.
3. While the spaghetti cooks, brown the sausage by breaking it up with a wooden spoon in a big skillet over medium-high heat.
4. Stir in the marinara sauce after adding it to the pan.
5. Combine the ricotta cheese, sliced mozzarella cheese, grated Parmesan cheese, salt, and pepper in a separate dish.
6. Add the cooked ziti noodles after draining in the same skillet as the sausage and marinara sauce.
7. To blend, stir.
8. A 9x13-inch baking dish should contain half of the pasta combination.
9. Pasta in the baking container should be covered with the ricotta cheese mixture.

10. Add the leftover pasta mixture on top.
11. Bake for 30 minutes with the foil covering the baking tray.
12. Remove the foil and continue baking for another 10 to 15 minutes, or until the top is bubbling and browned.
13. Before serving, allow settling for a short while.
14. If preferred, garnish with finely chopped fresh basil.

89. Grilled Shrimp Skewers with Mango Salsa

Ingredients:
- 1 lb large shrimp, peeled and deveined
- 1 tbsp. olive oil
- 1 tbsp. chili powder
- Salt and pepper, to taste
- Two mangoes, peeled and diced
- One small red onion, diced
- One small jalapeño pepper, seeded and minced
- 2 tbsp. chop fresh cilantro
- 2 tbsp. lime juice

Directions:
1. To medium-high heat, place the skillet or grill pan.
2. The shrimp, olive oil, chili powder, salt, and pepper should all be mixed together in one big serving dish.
3. Skewer the shrimp, leaving some room between each one.
4. 2 to 3 minutes on each side of the grill should be enough time to cook the shrimp spears completely.
5. Combine the mango cubes, red onion, jalapeo, cilantro, lime juice, and salt on a separate plate.

6. For added flavor, season the salsa with salt and pepper.
7. Serve the spicy shrimp spears with the mango salsa on the side.

Chapter 4:- Dessert Recipes

90.   Chocolate Chip Cookies

Ingredients:
- 1 cups of unsalted butter, softened
- 1 cups of white sugar
- 1 cups of brown sugar
- Two eggs
- 2 tsp. vanilla extract
- 3 cups of all-purpose flour
- 1 tsp. baking soda
- 1/2 tsp. salt
- 2 cups of semisweet chocolate chips

Directions:
1. A baking pan should be heated to 350°F (175°C).
2. A sizable basin should be used to incorporate butter, white sugar, and brown sugar fully.
3. After adding the vanilla extract, beat in each egg one at a time.
4. Flour, salt, and baking powder should be mixed together in a separate bowl.
5. Stirring constantly, gradually add the flour mixture to the butter mixture.
6. Stop adding flour once the two have been combined.

7. Put in the chocolate pieces and mix well.
8. By teaspoonfuls, drop the cookie batter onto an ungreased baking sheet.
9. The sides should brown after 8 to 10 minutes of baking.
10. After taking the cookies out of the oven, let them cool for a few minutes on the baking sheet before moving them to a metal cooling rack.

91.   Brownies

Ingredients:
- 1 cups of unsalted butter
- 2 1/4 cups of white sugar
- Four large eggs
- 1 1/4 cups of cocoa powder
- 1 tsp salt
- 1 tsp baking powder
- 1 tsp vanilla extract
- 1 1/2 cups of all-purpose flour
- 1 cups of semisweet chocolate chips

Instructions:
1. 350°F (180°C) should be the oven's temperature.
2. Mix the sugar and butter in a bowl until the mixture is fluffy.
3. Scramble the eggs one by one.
4. Combine salt, baking soda, vanilla extract, and chocolate powder.
5. Add the flour gradually while the wet ingredients are still being mixed.
6. Melt the chocolate and mix it in.

7. Pour the batter on a 9x13-inch baking sheet that has been buttered.
8. Put in the oven and bake for 25-30 minutes, checking frequently.
9. Relax and have fun!

92. Vanilla Cups ofcakes with Buttercream Frosting

Ingredients:
Cups ofcakes:

- 1/2 cups of unsalted butter, softened
- 1 cups of white sugar
- Two large eggs
- 1 tsp. vanilla extract
- 1 1/2 cups of all-purpose flour
- 1 3/4 tsp. baking powder
- 1/2 cups of milk

Buttercream frosting:

- 1/2 cups of unsalted butter, softened
- 2 cups of confectioners' sugar
- 1 tsp. vanilla extract
- 2-3 tbsp. milk

Directions:
Cups ofcakes:

1. A 12-cups of muffin pan should be lined with paper cups of. Set the oven's temperature to 350°F (175°C).

2. Combine the butter and sugar in a large mixing bowl and beat until fluffy.
3. Beat thoroughly after each addition of the yolks, one at a time.
4. Add the vanilla extract and stir.
5. Combine the baking powder and flour in a different dish.
6. Add the milk in small amounts while gradually adding the flour combination to the butter mixture, stirring until just combined.
7. Distribute the batter evenly among the muffin cups, filling them about halfway.
8. A toothpick put into the center of a cups ofcake should come out clean after baking it for 18 to 20 minutes.
9. Before frosting, remove from the oven and let cool thoroughly.

Buttercream frosting:

1. Beat the butter in a sizable mixing dish until it is smooth.
2. Add the confectioners' sugar gradually while beating until frothy and light.
3. Add the vanilla extract and stir.
4. One tbsp. At a time, gradually add the milk until the frosting has the required consistency.
5. The frosting can be piped or spread over the chilled cups ofcakes. Enjoy!

93.   Creme Brulee

Ingredients:

- 1-quart heavy cream
- One vanilla bean split lengthwise and scraped
- 1 cups of white sugar divided
- Six egg yolks

Directions:

1. The oven should be heated to 325°F (165°C).
2. In a medium saucepan, mix together the whole milk, vanilla bean and pulp, and a quarter of the sugar. The combination should be heated to a simmer over medium heat.
3. In a large bowl, mix together the extra sugar and the egg yolks.
4. Once the vanilla bean has been removed from the cream mixture, slowly pour the hot cream mixture into the egg yolks while whisking constantly.
5. Pour the mixture into a sizable measuring cups of or dish with a spout after passing it through a fine-mesh sieve.
6. In a sizable baking dish, put six 6-oz. ramekins. Fill each ramekin with the custard mixture, leaving a 1/4-inch area at the top.
7. Fill the baking dish with hot water until it reaches halfway up the sides of the ramekins.
8. Bake for 35-40 minutes, or until the custards are set but the centers are still jiggly.
9. The ramekins should be removed from the boiling water bath and the baking dish should be removed from the oven. Allow

the custards to settle to room temperature before chilling for at least two hours or up to three days in the refrigerator.

10.   Add a thin, even sugar coating to the top of each custard just before serving. Caramelize the sugar with a kitchen flame until crisp and golden brown. Quickly serve.

94.   Pecan Pie

Ingredients:

- One unbaked 9-inch pie crust
- Three eggs
- 1 cups of light corn syrup
- 1/2 cups of brown sugar
- 1/2 cups of granulated sugar
- 1/4 cups of unsalted butter, melted
- 1 tsp. vanilla extract
- 1/4 tsp. salt
- 1 1/2 cups of pecan halves

Directions:

1. 350°F (175°C) should be the oven's temperature.
2. In a large mixing bowl, thoroughly incorporate the eggs, corn syrup, brown sugar, granulated sugar, melted butter, vanilla extract, and salt.
3. Stir in the pecan half-shells.
4. The ingredients ought to be in the unbaked pie dough at this point.
5. Bake for 50 to 55 minutes to achieve a rosy surface and a firm interior.
6. Take out of oven and wait until it has cooled to cut and serve.

95.   Chocolate Truffles

Ingredients:
- 8 oz semisweet chocolate, chop
- 1/2 cups of heavy cream
- 2 tbsp unsalted butter at room temperature
- 1/4 cups of cocoa powder for rolling
- Optional toppings: chop nuts, shredded coconut, powdered sugar, or crushed cookies

Directions:
1. Put the chopped chocolate in a heat-resistant bowl and store it.
2. In a small pot over medium heat, the heavy cream needs to be heated until it simmers.
3. Wait one to two minutes before adding the warm cream to the chopped chocolate.
4. To ensure the chocolate is completely melted and the mixture is smooth, add the butter and stir.
5. After the ingredients have come to room temperature, wrap them in plastic and chill them for at least an hour, or until they have hardened.
6. Use a small spoon or melon baller to scoop out tiny amounts of the chocolate mixture, then use your hands to roll them into balls.
7. Before rolling the truffles in cocoa powder, coat them with your choice toppings.
8. Once the truffles have firmed up in the refrigerator, serve them.

96.   Raspberry Sorbet

Ingredients:

- 1 cups of granulated sugar
- 1 cups of water
- 4 cups of fresh raspberries
- 1 tbsp lemon juice

Directions:

1. Stirring occasionally, heat the sugar and water in a medium saucepan until the sugar is fully dissolved.
2. When you add the strawberries to the pan, make sure to mix them in.
3. The combination should simmer for 5 to 7 minutes or until it is thick and syrupy and the raspberries have broken down.
4. After turning off the heat, allow the combination to cool to room temperature.
5. Discard any solids as you strain the liquid into a blender using a fine-mesh strainer.
6. Blend the mixture along with the lemon juice until it is smooth.
7. Pour the mixture into an ice cream machine and process it as directed by the makers, or place it in a freezer-safe container and freeze it for two to three hours while stirring it every half-hour until it is firm.
8. Serve the sorbet right away by scooping it into bowls or cups of.

97. Coconut Macaroons

Ingredients:

- 2 1/2 cups of sweetened shredded coconut
- 2/3 cups of granulated sugar
- 1/4 cups of all-purpose flour
- 1/4 tsp salt
- Four egg whites
- 1 tsp vanilla extract

Directions:

1. The oven should be set to 325°F (165°C). Parchment paper should be used to line a baking sheet.
2. In a large dish, combine the sugar, flour, salt, and coconut flakes.
3. Egg whites and vanilla extract should be beaten separately until stiff peaks form.
4. Gently incorporate the egg whites into the coconut mixture until thoroughly combined.
5. Using a tiny cookie scoop or spoon, arrange the macaroons on the baking sheet as directed, spacing them about an inch apart.
6. Bake the macaroons for 20–25 minutes, or until they reach the desired firmness and golden color.
7. The macaroons must finish cooling on the baking sheet before being removed and served.

98.   Baked Alaska

Ingredients:
- 1-pint vanilla ice cream
- 1-pint strawberry ice cream
- 1-pint chocolate ice cream
- 1 (9-inch) round cake layer, baked and cooled
- Four egg whites
- 1/2 cups of granulated sugar

Directions:
1. Remove the ice cream from the refrigerator and let it sit at room temperature for 10 to 15 minutes to soften.
2. Cut a hole in the bottom of a 9-inch cake pan to fit the cake layer into a circle.
3. The layer cake should be positioned at the base of the baking dish.
4. Spread the vanilla ice cream over the cake layer using a large spoon or spatula and level it off.
5. As you repeat the procedure with the strawberry and chocolate ice cream layers, make sure each layer is even and homogeneous.
6. The cake topping and ice cream should be frozen for at least four hours.
7. The recommended oven temperature is 500 degrees Fahrenheit (260 degrees Celsius).
8. When the egg whites have been beaten in a large mixing bowl, they should be frothy.
9. The sugar should be added gradually while beating until stiff peaks form.

10. Turn the ice cream and cake layer onto a baking sheet covered with parchment paper after taking it out of the refrigerator.
11. Use a spatula or other flat object to create peaks and swirls after completely coating the ice cream and cake layer with the egg white mixture.
12. Put the Alaska on a baking sheet and bake for 2 to 3 minutes in the preheated oven, or until the meringue is golden.
13. Immediately serve.

99. Chocolate Cake

Ingredients:
- 2 cups of all-purpose flour
- 2 cups of white sugar
- 3/4 cups of cocoa powder
- 2 tsp baking powder
- 1 1/2 tsp baking soda
- 1 tsp salt
- 1 cups of milk
- 1/2 cups of vegetable oil
- Two large eggs
- 2 tsp vanilla extract
- 1 cups of boiling water

Instructions:
1. Set the oven's temperature to 350°F (180°C).
2. In a bowl, mix together the dry ingredients: flour, sugar, baking soda, baking powder, cocoa powder, and salt.

3. In a large bowl, whisk together the dry ingredients with the wet ingredients (milk, vegetable oil, eggs, and vanilla extract).
4. Blend thoroughly by beating.
5. Stir in hot water gradually.
6. Fill two greased 9-inch cake pans with the mixture.
7. Bake for 30–35 minutes, or until a toothpick inserted in the center comes out clean.
8. Relax and enjoy yourself!

100. Classic Apple Pie

Ingredients:
- One recipe for double-crust pie dough
- 6 cups of thinly sliced apples (about 6-7 medium apples)
- 2/3 cups of granulated sugar
- 3 tbsp all-purpose flour
- 1 tsp ground cinnamon
- 1/4 tsp ground nutmeg
- 1/4 tsp salt
- Two tbsp unsalted butter, cut into small pieces
- One egg, beaten

Directions:
1. Set the oven's temperature to 375°F (190°C).
2. To fit a 9-inch pie dish, roll out one side of the pie dough on a lightly dusted surface. Trim the sides of the dough before placing it in the pie dish.
3. Sliced apples, sugar, flour, cinnamon, nutmeg, and salt should all be combined in a big dish to coat the apples.

4. After adding the butter pieces to the top, pour the apple mixture into the pie crust that has been made.
5. Dust a clean work surface and roll out the remaining pie dough to fit the pie's top. Trim the corners of the dough before covering the filling.
6. A fork can be used to seal the pie's edges. Make slits in the pie's top so that steam can exit.
7. Over the pie's surface, brush the beaten egg.
8. Put the pie in the oven for 45-50 minutes, or until the crust is golden and the filling is bubbling.
9. Cool the pie completely before slicing and serving.

101. Chocolate Cake with Chocolate Frosting

Ingredients:
For the cake:

- 2 cups of all-purpose flour
- 2 cups of granulated sugar
- 3/4 cups of unsweetened cocoa powder
- 2 tsp baking powder
- 1 1/2 tsp baking soda
- 1 tsp salt
- 1 cups of milk
- 1/2 cups of vegetable oil
- Two eggs
- 2 tsp vanilla extract
- 1 cups of boiling water

For the frosting:

- 1/2 cups of unsalted butter, softened
- 2/3 cups of unsweetened cocoa powder
- 3 cups of powdered sugar
- 1/3 cups of milk
- 1 tsp vanilla extract

Directions:
1. 350°F (175°C) should be the oven's setting. Two 9-inch round cake dishes should be oiled and floured.
2. Add the dry ingredients (flour, sugar, baking soda, salt, baking powder, and cocoa powder) to a large bowl and stir to combine.
3. Mix the milk, oil, eggs, and vanilla extract together in a mixer. 2 minutes of medium-speed beating.
4. The hot water needs to be stirred in completely. There won't be much of a mixture.
5. Distribute the batter evenly between the cake pans.
6. A toothpick inserted into the center of the cakes after 30–35 minutes of baking should come out clean.
7. Ten minutes should pass after the cakes are removed from the pans so they can cool completely on wire racks.
8. Softened butter is creamed with an electric mixer on medium speed to make the frosting.
9. Both cocoa powder and powdered sugar are added and beaten into the mixture.
10. Add the milk and vanilla extract once the frosting is creamy and smooth, and beat at a medium-high speed until mixed.
11. Place one tier of the cakes on a serving plate and generously top it once the cakes have chilled completely.

12. The top and sides of the cake should be covered with any remaining frosting before adding the second cake on top.

13. It is best to serve the cake soon away.

102. Strawberry Shortcake

Ingredients:

- 2 cups of all-purpose flour
- 2 tsp baking powder
- 1/2 tsp baking soda
- 1/4 tsp salt
- 1/2 cups of unsalted butter, softened
- 1 cups of granulated sugar
- Two large eggs
- 1 tsp vanilla extract
- 1/2 cups of whole milk
- 1 cups of whipped cream
- 2 cups of fresh strawberries, sliced

Instructions:

1. Activate the 375°F oven.
2. In a medium bowl, whisk together the flour, salt, baking soda, and baking powder.
3. In a separate dish, fluffy butter and sugar are combined.
4. After adding the vanilla extract, add the eggs one at a time.
5. While steadily stirring until just incorporated, add the milk to the flour mixture.
6. A toothpick placed in the center of the cake should come out clean after baking for 25 to 30 minutes in a greased 9-inch cake pan.

7. The chilled cake needs to have sliced strawberries and sweetened cream added.

103. Tiramisu

Ingredients:
- Six egg yolks
- 3/4 cups of granulated sugar
- 2/3 cups of milk
- 1 1/4 cups of heavy cream
- 1/2 tsp vanilla extract
- 1 lb mascarpone cheese, room temperature
- 2 cups of strong brewed coffee, cooled
- 1/4 cups of rum or brandy
- 24-30 ladyfingers
- cocoa powder for dusting

Instructions:
1. Carefully combine the sugar and egg yolks in a large mixing dish while lightening the color.
2. Mix in the milk entirely after adding it.
3. Cooking the combination over medium heat while stirring continuously should cause the mixture to thicken and coat the back of a spoon. (about 10-15 minutes).
4. Let the food cool to room temperature after removing it from the flames.
5. Heavy cream and vanilla extract are beaten to stiff peaks in a separate bowl.
6. In a separate large dish, thoroughly blend the mascarpone cheese.

7. Whipping cream is incorporated into the cooled egg mixture before adding the mascarpone cheese.
8. In a tiny bowl, combine coffee and cognac or rum.
9. After dipping the ladyfingers in the coffee concoction, arrange them in a layer at the bottom of a 9x13-inch dish.
10. Repeat with another layer of moistened ladyfingers and the remaining mascarpone mixture.
11. Refrigerate, covered, for at least three hours and up to overnight.
12. I cover the food with cocoa powder before serving.

104. Chocolate Mousse

Ingredients:
- 8 oz semisweet chocolate, chop
- 1/4 cups of unsalted butter, softened
- Four eggs separated
- 1/4 cups of granulated sugar
- 1/2 tsp vanilla extract
- 1/2 cups of heavy cream
- Whipped cream and chocolate shavings for garnish

Instructions:
1. Use a double boiler or a microwave to smooth out the chocolate thoroughly.
2. The butter is added, and then it is stirred.
3. The egg yolks should be fluffy and light in color. Combine sugar, vanilla essence, and another dish.
4. Before adding the cocoa mixture, stir everything thoroughly.

5. Egg whites should be whisked until stiff peaks form and placed in a separate bowl.
6. To achieve soft peaks, rich milk must be whisked.
7. The cream and egg whites should be whipped, then gently folded into the chocolate.
8. Serve chilled, after chilling the mixture for at least an hour in serving glasses.
9. Whipping cream and chocolate bits can be added as a garnish before serving.

105. Apple Crisp

Ingredients:
- 6 cups of apples, peeled, cored, and sliced
- 1/2 cups of all-purpose flour
- 1/2 cups of brown sugar
- 1/2 cups of rolled oats
- 1/2 cups of unsalted butter, softened
- 1 tsp ground cinnamon
- 1/2 tsp ground nutmeg
- 1/4 tsp salt
- Vanilla ice cream

Instructions:
1. Set the oven to 375 degrees.
2. Prepare a 9-by-9-inch baking dish by arranging the apple slices in a single layer.
3. Flour, brown sugar, rolled oats, butter, cinnamon, nutmeg, and salt should be combined in a separate bowl.

4. With a fork or pastry blender, combine the ingredients until they resemble crumbs.
5. Distribute the mixture equally over the apples.
6. Bake for 45 minutes at 350 degrees until the apples are soft and the topping is golden brown.
7. Put a scoop of vanilla ice cream on top and serve warm.

106. Carrot Cake with Cream Cheese Frosting

Ingredients:
- 2 cups of all-purpose flour
- 2 tsp baking powder
- 1 tsp baking soda
- 1 tsp ground cinnamon
- 1/2 tsp ground nutmeg
- 1/2 tsp salt
- 1 1/2 cups of granulated sugar
- 1 cups of vegetable oil
- Three large eggs
- 2 cups of grated carrots
- 1/2 cups of chop walnuts
- 8 oz cream cheese, softened
- 1/4 cups of unsalted butter, softened
- 2 cups of powdered sugar
- 1 tsp vanilla extract

Instructions:

1. While your oven is heating to 350 degrees Fahrenheit, prepare your two 9-inch cake pans by cleaning, dusting, and oiling them.
2. Combine the flour, salt, cinnamon, nutmeg, baking soda, and flour in a medium bowl.
3. The oil and sugar should be thoroughly mixed in a large bowl. Whip the mixture well after each addition of an egg.
4. Blend after each addition as you progressively add the flour mixture. Stirring, add the chop pecans and carrots that have been shredded.
5. After 25 to 30 minutes in the oven, the cakes should be done when tested with a toothpick in the center. Fill the prepped cake pans with the batter.
6. Ten minutes should pass while the cakes cool in the pans before being transferred to a wire stand to complete cooling.
7. To make the icing, cream cheese and butter must be thoroughly beaten. The vanilla essence and powdered sugar should be added gradually and thoroughly combined.
8. Decorate the dessert following its serving.

107. Chocolate Pudding

Ingredients:

- 2 cups of whole milk
- 1/2 cups of granulated sugar
- 1/4 cups of cornstarch
- 1/4 cups of unsweetened cocoa powder
- 1/4 tsp salt

- Two large egg yolks
- 2 tbsp unsalted butter, softened
- 1 tsp vanilla extract
- Whipped cream and chocolate shavings for garnish

Instructions:
1. In a medium pot, stir the milk, sugar, cornstarch, cocoa powder, and salt until thoroughly combined.
2. To thicken the liquid, bring it to a boil while stirring constantly.
3. The egg yolks should be beaten together in a separate bowl until light and airy.
4. The hot milk mixture should be whisked steadily into the egg whites in about 1 cups of.
5. Returning the egg mixture to the pan, stir continuously for 2 minutes over medium heat or until the pudding thickens and bubbles.
6. The pan is thoroughly mixed after adding the butter and vanilla extract.
7. Put the custard in individual bowls and chill them in the fridge for at least an hour before serving.
8. Add chocolate crumbs and whipped cream as a garnish before serving.

108. Key Lime Pie

Ingredients:

- 1 1/2 cups of graham cracker crumbs
- 6 tbsp unsalted butter, melted
- 1/3 cups of granulated sugar
- Three large egg yolks
- 14 oz can of sweetened condensed milk
- 1/2 cups of key lime juice
- 1 tbsp lime zest
- Whipped cream and lime slices for garnish

Instructions:

1. Preheat oven to 375 degrees F. Crumbs of graham crackers, sugar, and warmed butter should be combined in a medium dish.
2. Combine all ingredients in a pie dish 9 inches in diameter and roast for ten to twelve minutes. Wait a while for the components to settle down.
3. Egg whites should be beaten in a big dish until they become dense and creamy.
4. It's essential to thoroughly combine everything before adding the condensed milk.
5. Mix the lime juice and rind before adding more.
6. After 10 to 12 minutes of baking, the filling should be solid, at which point you can pour it into the prepared shell.
7. After an hour at ambient temperature in the refrigerator, the pie will be ready to serve.
8. Serve with whipped topping and lemon wedges.

109. Chocolate Chip Banana Bread

Ingredients:

- 2 cups of all-purpose flour
- 1 tsp baking soda
- 1/2 tsp salt
- 1/2 cups of unsalted butter, softened
- 3/4 cups of brown sugar
- Two large eggs
- 1 tsp vanilla extract
- Three ripe bananas, mashed
- 1 cups of semisweet chocolate chips

Instructions:

1. For a temperature of 350 degrees in the oven, get ready. Get ready in a 9-by-5-by-3-inch oiled bread container.
2. In a medium bowl, combine the flour, baking powder, and salt.
3. Butter and brown sugar should be creamed together in a large dish using a mixer set to medium speed until light and frothy.
4. It's important to add the vanilla extract and eggs separately.
5. Bananas, once mashed, can be introduced afterward.
6. Add the flour combination to the bowl and whisk slowly until combined.
7. Mix in the pieces of chocolate.
8. Bake for 50–60 minutes, or until a knife stuck in the middle comes out clear, after dumping the mixture into the prepped bread pan.

9. After letting the bread rest for 10 minutes in the skillet, transfer it to a metal stand to finish chilling.

110. Peach Cobbler

Ingredients:

- 6 cups of peeled and sliced peaches
- 1/2 cups of granulated sugar
- 1/4 cups of brown sugar
- 1 tsp ground cinnamon
- 1/4 tsp ground nutmeg
- 2 tbsp cornstarch
- 1/4 cups of unsalted butter, melted
- 1 cups of all-purpose flour
- 1/4 cups of granulated sugar
- 1 tsp baking powder
- 1/2 tsp salt
- 3/4 cups of milk

Instructions:

1. The oven temperature is set to 375 degrees. The baking dish needs to be 9 inches on a side at least.
2. Peaches, granulated sugar, brown sugar, cinnamon, nutmeg, and cornstarch should all be combined in a large bowl and mixed thoroughly.
3. The prepared baking dish must now contain the equally distributed melted butter.
4. Spread the butter over the fruit topping.
5. In another basin, combine the flour, sugar, baking soda, and salt.

6. Add the milk and completely blend.
7. The batter should be evenly strewn over the peaches.
8. When the peaches are boiling, and the top is golden brown, wait 45 to 50 minutes before serving.
9. Cool the food for at least 10 minutes before serving.

111. Cherry Pie

Ingredients:
- One double pie crust recipe
- 4 cups of pitted cherries, fresh or frozen
- 1/2 cups of granulated sugar
- 1/4 cups of cornstarch
- 1 tsp vanilla extract
- 1/4 tsp almond extract
- One tbsp unsalted butter, cut into small pieces
- One egg, beaten (for egg wash)
- Coarse sugar (for sprinkling)

Instructions:
1. Turn on the 375°F oven.
2. Roll out one of the pie crusts and fit it into a 9-inch pie dish.
3. In a large bowl, mix together the cherries, sugar, cornstarch, vanilla extract, and almond extract.
4. Spread cherry filling over pie crust.
5. The tiny bits of butter should be scattered over the cherry mixture's top.
6. The second pie crust should be rolled out and cut into pieces.
7. Make a latticework pattern with the pie crust strips and arrange them over the cherry filling.

8. Coat the lattice in egg wash, and then sprinkle coarse sugar on top.

9. To get a boiling middle and a golden brown exterior, bake for 50–55 minutes.

10. Before serving, allow chilling for at least 30 minutes.

112. Peanut Butter Cups of

Ingredients:
- 1 cups of creamy peanut butter
- 1/2 cups of unsalted butter, softened
- 1/2 cups of confectioners' sugar
- 1/2 tsp vanilla extract
- 1/4 tsp salt
- 2 cups of semisweet chocolate chips

Instructions:
1. Use paper liners to fill a muffin pan.
2. In a medium bowl, beat the peanut butter and melted butter together until smooth.
3. Mix thoroughly after adding the salt, vanilla essence, and confectioners' sugar.
4. More petite balls of the concoction should be formed, and each one should be pressed into the bottom of a paper liner in a muffin pan.
5. Melt the chocolate chunks in a microwave-safe bowl, stirring every 20 seconds.
6. Each paper cup should have melted chocolate drizzled on top of the peanut butter mixture.

7. After at least 30 minutes in the fridge, the chocolate should have hardened.
8. The peanut butter cakes should be stored in the refrigerator in a sealed receptacle until ready to serve.

113. Rice Pudding

Ingredients:
- 1 cups of white rice, rinsed and drained
- 2 cups of water
- 2 cups of whole milk
- 1/2 cups of granulated sugar
- 1/4 tsp salt
- One cinnamon stick
- 1 tsp vanilla extract
- 1/2 cups of raisins
- Ground cinnamon (for garnish)

Instructions:
1. Rice, water, and a cinnamon stick should be combined in a medium saucepan.
2. Once the mixture reaches a boil, reduce the heat to low and cover the skillet.
3. When the rice is soft and all the water has been absorbed, after 18-20 minutes, it is done.
4. Sugar, salt, vanilla extract, and milk can be added to the rice while it cooks.
5. Cook, stirring frequently, until the mixture reaches a boil over medium heat.

6. Cook the mixture for 25-30 minutes over medium heat or until it reaches the desired thickness.
7. The cinnamon stalk must be removed before using raisins.
8. Serve warm, cold, or at room temperature, and sprinkle with ground cinnamon.

114. Chocolate Covered Strawberries

Ingredients:
- 1 lb fresh strawberries, washed and dried
- 8 oz semisweet chocolate chips
- 2 tbsp vegetable shortening

Instructions:
1. Use parchment paper to cover a baking sheet.
2. In a double boiler or microwave-safe bowl, melt the vegetable shortening and chocolate chips together.
3. Swirl the melted chocolate over the strawberries while holding them by the stalk.
4. Onto the prepared baking tray, put the coated strawberries.
5. The leftover strawberries should be used next.
6. Refrigerate the strawberries for at least 15 minutes or until the chocolate has hardened.
7. Dispense and savor!

115. Red Velvet Cake

Ingredients:
For the cake:

- 2 1/2 cups of all-purpose flour
- 1 1/2 cups of granulated sugar
- 1 tsp baking soda
- 1 tsp salt
- 1 tsp cocoa powder
- 1 1/2 cups of vegetable oil
- 1 cups of buttermilk, room temperature
- Two large eggs, room temperature
- 1 oz red food coloring
- 1 tsp vanilla extract
- 1 tsp white vinegar

For the cream cheese frosting:

- 8 oz cream cheese, room temperature
- 1/2 cups of unsalted butter, room temperature
- 4 cups of powdered sugar
- 1 tsp vanilla extract

Instructions:
1. Set the oven to 350°F. Two 9-inch cake pans should be greased and have parchment paper on the bases.
2. Combine the dry ingredients (flour, sugar, baking soda, salt, and cocoa powder) in a large bowl.
3. Whisk the oil, buttermilk, eggs, food coloring, vanilla essence, and vinegar in a separate bowl.

4. Mix the dry ingredients just until mixed after adding the wet ingredients.
5. Evenly distribute the batter among the prepped pans.
6. After 30–35 minutes in the oven, test the cake by inserting a toothpick in the center; it should come out clean.
7. Let the cakes finish cooling in their containers.
8. Cream cheese and butter should be combined and thoroughly beaten to create the icing.
9. Add the powdered sugar and vanilla essence gradually while beating until fluffy.
10. Put one layer on a serving dish or cake stand after the cakes have cooled completely.
11. Place the second cake layer on top of the frosted first.
12. Use the leftover frosting to cover the complete cake.
13. Dispense and savor!

116. Blueberry Muffins

Ingredients:
- 2 cups of all-purpose flour
- 1 tbsp baking powder
- 1/2 tsp salt
- 1/2 cups of unsalted butter, softened
- 1 cups of granulated sugar
- Two large eggs
- 1/2 cups of whole milk
- 1 tsp vanilla extract
- 1 1/2 cups of fresh blueberries

Instructions:

1. Paper liners should cover a muffin pan as the oven is preheated to 375°F (190°C).
2. Sift the flour, baking powder, and salt into a bowl of suitable size.
3. In a large dish, light and creamy butter and sugar can be achieved by beating them together for two to three minutes.
4. Each egg should be added separately and thoroughly blended in before the next.
5. Add the vanilla extract and milk to the large bowl. Mix the two together.
6. The dry components should be added gradually to the large bowl and combined just until combined.
7. Blueberries should be added and mixed.
8. Divide the batter evenly among the muffin cups, filling them about halfway.
9. A toothpick put into the center of a muffin should come out clean after 20 to 25 minutes of baking.
10. Before transferring the muffins to a wire tray to finish cooling, give them a few minutes to cool in the pan.

117. Peanut Butter Cookies

Ingredients:

- 1/2 cups of unsalted butter, softened
- 1/2 cups of granulated sugar
- 1/2 cups of brown sugar
- 1/2 cups of creamy peanut butter
- One large egg

- 1 tsp vanilla extract
- 1 1/4 cups of all-purpose flour
- 1/2 tsp baking powder
- 1/2 tsp baking soda
- 1/4 tsp salt

Instructions:

1. In order to prepare, line a baking sheet with parchment paper and preheat the oven to 350 degrees Fahrenheit (180 degrees Celsius).
2. Mix the peanut butter, powdered sugar, brown sugar, and butter in a large bowl. Beat for two to three minutes.
3. In the large dish, combine the egg and vanilla extract. Ensure that the flavors blend well.
4. In another dish, mash together the all-purpose flour, baking soda, baking powder, and salt.
5. Mix well after each addition as you add the dry ingredients to the large dish.
6. Place the dough balls on the prepared baking sheet at a distance of 2 inches apart.
7. Carefully flatten each disc into a crossing pattern using the fork's tines.
8. Three hundred fifty degrees should be used for baking, and the oven should be on for between 10 and 12 minutes.
9. Once the biscuits have cooled for a few minutes on the baking sheet, transfer them to a metal stand to chill completely.

118. Cheesecake with Raspberry Sauce

Ingredients:
Cheesecake:

- 2 cups of graham cracker crumbs
- 1/4 cups of sugar
- 1/2 cups of unsalted butter, melted
- Four packages (8 oz each) of cream cheese at room temperature
- 1 1/4 cups of sugar
- 1 tsp vanilla extract
- Four eggs
- 1/3 cups of heavy cream

Raspberry sauce:

- 2 cups of fresh or frozen raspberries
- 1/2 cups of sugar
- 1/4 cups of water
- 1 tbsp cornstarch

Instructions:
1. One hundred sixty-five degrees Celsius must be reached in the oven. A greased and stored 9-inch spring form plate is ready for use.
2. Graham cracker crumbs, sugar, and melted butter should all be mixed together in a bowl. Press the ingredients into the bottom and up the edges of the prepared skillet to create a rim. Put it in the oven for 8-10 minutes, or until it just starts

to turn a light color. Please dispose of the heat source until it has cooled.

3. Blend cream cheese, sugar, and vanilla in a big bowl. One egg at a time, properly blending in between additions, should be added. Thoroughly blend the heavy cream.

4. When the filling has cooled, spread it evenly over the crust using a spoon. Wait 45-50 minutes in the oven for the center to be set and the edges to start browning. Please dispose of the heat source until it has cooled.

5. Make the raspberry sauce while you wait for the cheesecake to set. In a small pot, mix the strawberries, water, and sugar. Cooking the mixture over medium heat while stirring occasionally should cause the blackberries to break down and the mixture to somewhat thicken. Carefully combine the cornmeal and cool water in a small bowl. The raspberry syrup should be combined with the condensed cornflour mixture by whisking them together. The fire needs to be extinguished and given time to die down.

6. Once it has chilled, the cheesecake is prepared to be taken out of the skillet and put on a serving plate. Sprinkle some raspberry sauce on top just before serving.

119. Lemon Bars

Ingredients:

- 1 cups of unsalted butter, softened
- 1/2 cups of powdered sugar
- 2 cups of all-purpose flour
- Four large eggs
- 1 1/2 cups of granulated sugar
- 1/4 cups of all-purpose flour
- 1/2 tsp. baking powder
- 1/4 tsp. salt
- 1/3 cups of fresh lemon juice
- 1 tbsp. lemon zest
- Powdered sugar for dusting

Instructions:

1. The oven to 350 degrees Fahrenheit. A 9x13-inch pastry pan should be greased.
2. Butter and powdered sugar should be creamed together in a big dish until light and fluffy.
3. Flour should be added gradually and mixed just enough.
4. Bake the combination, pressed into the baking dish as directed, for 18 to 20 minutes or until golden brown.
5. In the meantime, combine the eggs, granulated sugar, flour, baking soda, salt, lemon juice, and lemon zest in a separate big dish.
6. After spreading the lemon mixture over the baked crust, put the skillet back in the oven.
7. The filling must be baked for 20 to 25 minutes to set.
8. Allow the bars to finish cooling in the skillet.

9. Cut into squares and sprinkle with sugar once completely cold.

120. Oatmeal Raisin Cookies

Ingredients:
- 1 cups of unsalted butter, softened
- 1 cups of granulated sugar
- 1 cups of brown sugar
- Two large eggs
- 2 tsp. vanilla extract
- 1 1/2 cups of all-purpose flour
- 1 tsp. baking soda
- 1 tsp. cinnamon
- 1/2 tsp. salt
- 3 cups of old-fashioned oats
- 1 cups of raisins

Instructions:
1. The oven to 350 degrees Fahrenheit. Spread parchment paper on a baking sheet.
2. In a large bowl, cream the butter and sugars together until fluffy.
3. Incorporate the eggs and vanilla essence after adding them.
4. Mix the flour, baking soda, cinnamon, and salt in a separate dish.
5. Mix until just mixed after gradually incorporating the flour mixture into the butter mixture.
6. Add the raisins and grains after that.

7. To place the mixture on the preheated baking sheet, use a cookie scoop or spoon and space the drops about 2 inches apart.
8. Wait 12 to 15 minutes in the oven, or until the edges start to brown.
9. After five minutes, transfer the biscuits to a wire cooling rack to finish cooling.

Chapter 5:- Snacks Recipes

121. Trail Mix

Ingredients:
- 1 cups of almonds
- 1 cups of cashews
- 1 cups of pumpkin seeds
- 1 cups of dried cranberries
- 1 cups of dark chocolate chips

Instructions:
1. Three hundred fifty degrees Fahrenheit in the oven.
2. Place the almonds, cashews, and pumpkin seeds on a baking sheet.
3. Brown the sugars in a hot oven for 10 to 12 minutes.
4. Wait for it to cool down after you take it out of the oven.
5. Combine the dried cranberries, dark chocolate, and dark chocolate chunks with the pumpkin seeds in a bowl.
6. The trail mix will keep for up to two weeks if stored properly.

122. Homemade Granola Bars

Ingredients:

- 2 cups of old-fashioned rolled oats
- 1/2 cups of honey
- 1/2 cups of creamy peanut butter
- 1/4 cups of chocolate chips
- 1/4 cups of chop almonds
- 1/4 cups of dried cranberries

Instructions:

1. Three hundred fifty degrees Fahrenheit in the oven.
2. Thoroughly mix the oats, honey, and peanut butter in a large bowl.
3. Add the chopped almonds, chocolate bits, and dried cranberries. Completely combine.
4. In a 9x13-inch baking dish, press the mixture down using oiled hands.
5. Wait 20–25 minutes, or until the top is browned, before serving.
6. Once the bars have cooled completely, they can be cut.
7. Stored properly, granola bars have a shelf life of up to a week.

123. Fruit Salad

Ingredients:

- 2 cups of strawberries, chop
- 2 cups of blueberries
- 2 cups of pineapple, chop
- 1 cups of kiwi, chop

- 1 cups of grapes
- 1/4 cups of honey
- 2 tbsp. Of fresh lime juice

Instructions:
1. Combine the strawberries, blueberries, pineapple, kiwi, and grapes in a big dish.
2. Mix the honey and fresh lime juice in a small dish.
3. Mix the honey and lime juice combination well before adding it to the fruit salad.
4. Offer cold.

124. Popcorn with Seasoning

Ingredients:
- 1/2 cups of popcorn kernels
- 2 tbsp. of vegetable oil
- 1/4 cups of butter, melted
- 1 tbsp. of nutritional yeast
- 1/2 tsp. of smoked paprika
- 1/2 tsp. of garlic powder
- 1/2 tsp. of onion powder
- 1/4 tsp. of cayenne pepper
- Salt to taste

Instructions:
1. Vegetable oil should be heated on medium-high in a large saucepan.
2. Add the pieces of popcorn and cover them with a lid.
3. Repeat this process until the popping stops.

4. Popcorn is removed from the heat and placed in a big dish.
5. Melted butter, nutritional yeast, smoked paprika, garlic powder, onion powder, cayenne pepper, and salt should all be combined in a small dish.
6. After the butter has melted, sprinkle the popcorn with the seasonings and toss to coat.
7. Quickly serve.

125. Vegetable Chips

Ingredients:
- One bunch of kale
- One beet
- One sweet potato
- 2 tbsp. of olive oil
- Salt and pepper to taste

Instructions:
1. The oven should be heated to 350°F (175°C).
2. All of the kale stems, beet, and sweet potato need to be cleaned and dried before you begin.
3. Cut the sweet potato and beet into thin slices.
4. The kale leaves should be stripped of their tough stem and torn into bite-sized chunks.
5. Olive oil, salt, and pepper should be mixed with the veggies.
6. Spread the vegetables out in a single layer on a baking sheet.
7. Turn the chips over halfway through baking and bake for 15 to 20 minutes.
8. Quickly serve.

126. Hummus and Pita Chips

Ingredients:

- Two cans of chickpeas, drained and rinsed
- 1/4 cups of tahini
- 1/4 cups of lemon juice
- Two garlic cloves minced
- 2 tbsp. of olive oil
- Salt and pepper to taste
- Pita bread sliced into triangles

Instructions:

1. Blend the beans, tahini, lemon juice, garlic, extra virgin olive oil, salt, and pepper in a food processor.
2. Taste the seasoning and make any required adjustments.
3. Pita crackers should be served with the hummus.
4. Make sure your oven is preheated to 375 degrees F (190 degrees C) before you begin making the pita crumbs.
5. Place the pita bread pieces in a single layer on a baking sheet.
6. Olive oil is rubbed over the focaccia, then salt is added.
7. Cook until crisp and golden, 10 to 12 minutes.
8. Quickly serve with hummus.

127. Sweet Potato Fries

Ingredients:

- Two large sweet potatoes
- 2 tbsp cornstarch
- 2 tbsp olive oil
- 1/2 tsp paprika
- 1/2 tsp garlic powder
- 1/2 tsp salt
- 1/4 tsp black pepper

Instructions:

1. The oven should be set to 425 °F (220 °C).
2. Sweet potatoes need to be washed and peeled. Separate them into pieces of similar length.
3. Over the beautiful potato pieces in a large basin, sprinkle the cornstarch. Toss to coat.
4. Toss the sweet potato sticks with the olive oil so that they are evenly coated.
5. In a small dish, combine paprika, garlic powder, salt, and black pepper.
6. The sweet potato sticks should be liberally seasoned.
7. Line a baking sheet with parchment paper and arrange the sweet potato sticks in a single layer.
8. When the sweet potato fries are crisp and golden brown, bake them for 20 to 25 minutes, flipping them halfway through.
9. The dish should be served at room temperature, so take it out of the oven now. Enjoy!

128. Toast with Avocado and Egg

Ingredients:
- Two slices of bread
- One ripe avocado
- Two eggs
- Salt and pepper
- Olive oil or butter for cooking

Instructions:
1. Toast the bread as you like it.
2. As the bread toasts, cut the avocado in half and remove the pit. The meat should be removed and mashed in a small bowl with a utensil—season with salt and pepper to taste.
3. Medium heat in a Teflon pan with a splash of olive oil or a pat of butter.
4. Season the eggs with salt and pepper once they have been broken into the pan. Two to three minutes should do it; you want the whites to be set but the eggs to be soft.
5. The toast would have benefited from having avocado smeared on it before the eggs were added. Quickly dish it out.

129. Guacamole

Ingredients:
- Three ripe avocados
- 1/4 cups of diced onion
- 1/4 cups of diced tomato
- 1 tbsp. chop cilantro
- 1 tbsp. lime juice

- Salt and pepper to taste

Instructions:

1. Remove the pit from the avocados, then scoop the meat into a bowl.
2. Mash the avocado with a spatula until it reaches the desired smoothness. (chunky or smooth).
3. Mix well before adding the chop tomato, onion, and parsley.
4. Add lime juice and season to flavor with salt and pepper.
5. Make sure everything is well combined.
6. Check the flavor and adjust the seasoning if necessary.
7. Serve quickly as a side dish, on top of tacos or fajitas, or with tortilla chips.

130. Homemade Hummus

Ingredients:

- One can (15 oz) chickpeas (garbanzo beans), drained and rinsed
- 1/4 cups of tahini (sesame seed paste)
- 2-3 cloves garlic, minced
- 3 tbsp. extra-virgin olive oil
- 3 tbsp. lemon juice
- 1/4 tsp. ground cumin
- Salt and pepper to taste
- Water (as needed for consistency)

Instructions:

1. The legumes should be processed in a food processor to a fine mash.

2. Throw some tahini, garlic, olive oil, lemon juice, cumin, salt, and pepper into a food processor and blend until smooth..
3. The mixture should be homogeneous.
4. Add water (one tbsp. at a time) to achieve the required consistency if the hummus is too thick.
5. Check the flavor and adjust the seasoning if necessary.
6. Put the hummus in a dish and top it with some olive oil.
7. Serve as a dip with crackers, pita, vegetables, or in sandwiches.

131. Caprese Skewers

Ingredients:
- Cherry or grape tomatoes
- Fresh mozzarella cheese
- Fresh basil leaves
- Balsamic vinegar
- Olive oil
- Salt and pepper
- Skewers

Instructions:
1. Basil stems and tomatoes should be cleaned and dried.
2. Cut the mozzarella cheese into bite-sized pieces.
3. A cherry tomato, a slice of mozzarella cheese, and a basil leaf should be strung onto a skewer.
4. Repeat the technique with the remaining parts to create as many skewers as you need.
5. Place the skewers in a line on a serving platter.
6. Toss the spears in a mixture of olive oil and balsamic vinegar.

7. Season the food with salt and pepper to taste.

8. Serve as a starter or refreshment immediately away.

132. Bruschetta

Ingredients:

- One large baguette of Italian bread sliced into 1/2-inch thick slices
- 4-5 ripe tomatoes, diced
- 3-4 cloves garlic, minced
- 1/4 cups of chopped fresh basil
- 2 tbsp. extra-virgin olive oil
- Salt and pepper to taste
- Balsamic vinegar

Instructions:

1. Set the oven to 400°F.
2. Put the bread cubes in a single layer on an oiled baking sheet and bake.
3. For about 5-7 minutes, bake the bread in the oven or until crisp and browned.
4. In a serving dish, mix together the tomato dice, basil leaves, garlic cloves, olive oil, salt, and pepper.
5. Pour some balsamic vinegar over the tomato mixture, if preferred.
6. Spread the tomato sauce on the toasted bread cubes.

133. Deviled Eggs

Ingredients:

- Six hard-boiled eggs
- 1/4 cups of mayonnaise
- 1 tsp. Dijon mustard
- 1/2 tsp. white vinegar
- 1/8 tsp. salt
- Pinch of black pepper
- Paprika or fresh herbs for garnish

Instructions:

1. The hard-boiled eggs should be peeled and split longitudinally.
2. The egg yolks should be removed and put in a small mixing dish.
3. With a fork, mash the eggs until they are crumbly.
4. When you add the mayonnaise, Dijon mustard, white vinegar, salt, and pepper, you should blend it until it's smooth.
5. Fill a plastic bag with the corner cut off or a piping bag with the yolk concoction.
6. The combination should be piped into the egg-white halves.
7. For decoration, add paprika or fresh herbs.
8. Refrigerate the deviled eggs for at least 30 minutes before serving.

134. Mini Quiches

Ingredients:

- 1 1/2 cups of all-purpose flour
- 1/2 tsp. salt
- 1/2 cups of (1 stick) unsalted butter, chilled and cut into small pieces
- 2-3 tbsp. ice water
- 1/2 cups of chop cooked ham, bacon, or spinach
- 1/2 cups of shredded cheddar cheese
- Three large eggs
- 1 cups of heavy cream
- Salt and pepper to taste
- Nonstick cooking spray

Instructions:

1. The oven should be preheated at 375°F (190°C).
2. Combine the flour and salt in a large bowl and stir to combine.
3. Use a pastry blender to cut in the cooled butter until the dough resembles coarse crumbs.
4. Add another spoonful once the dough becomes a ball, and continue mixing in the ice water.
5. On a lightly floured surface, roll the dough out to a thickness of about 1/8 inch.
6. Cut out tiny circles from the dough using a glass or a biscuit machine.
7. Push a dough disk into each cups of after lightly spraying a miniature muffin pan with nonstick cooking spray.

8. Add shredded cheddar cheese, chopped ham, bacon, or spinach to the muffin cups of.
9. Whisk the eggs and the heavy cream together in a separate mixing bowl. Pepper and salt it for flavor.
10. The egg mixture should be poured into each muffin cups of until about 3/4 full.
11. If you want a golden crust and a set egg filling, bake the mini quiches for 20 to 25 minutes.
12. Allow settling for a brief period before serving.

135. Cheese Plate

Ingredients:
- Assorted cheeses (choose a variety of types, such as soft, complex, and blue cheese)
- Crackers or bread
- Fresh or dried fruit
- Nuts
- Olives or pickles
- Honey or jam

Instructions:
1. Pick a range of cheeses, such as blue, gouda, cheddar, and brie. For a good variety, it's best to have at least three various kinds of cheese.
2. Place the cheeses in a row on a sizable plate or wooden board, leaving room between each one for the fixings.
3. Place crackers or bread around the cheese on the plate.
4. Fruit can be added to the plate, and fresh or dried fruits such as grapes, figs, or dried apricots can be added.

5. Add nuts to the dish, like almonds or walnuts.
6. Include pickles or olives on the plate.
7. Add honey or jam to the platter for a sweet counterpoint to the salty cheese.
8. For the best flavor, serve the cheese platter at room temperature after letting it come to room temperature.

136. Buffalo Chicken Dip

Ingredients:
- 2 cups of cooked and shredded chicken
- 8 oz cream cheese, softened
- 1/2 cups of buffalo sauce
- 1/2 cups of ranch dressing
- 1/2 cups of shredded cheddar cheese
- 1/4 cups of crumbled blue cheese
- Green onions, chop
- Tortilla chips or celery sticks for serving

Instructions:
1. 350°F (175°C) should be the oven's setting.
2. Add cooked and shredded chicken, cream cheese, buffalo sauce, ranch dressing, cheddar cheese, and crumbled blue cheese in a sizable mixing bowl.
3. Coat a baking sheet with the batter.
4. Wait 20-25 minutes in the oven for the cheese to melt and bubble.
5. Finely chopped green scallions should be used to decorate it after removing it from the oven.
6. Serve hot with tortilla chips or stalks of celery.

137. Spinach Artichoke Dip

Ingredients:
- 8 oz cream cheese, softened
- 1/2 cups of sour cream
- 1/2 cups of mayonnaise
- 1/2 cups of grated Parmesan cheese
- 1/2 cups of shredded mozzarella cheese
- One can (14 oz) of artichoke hearts, drained and chopped
- 1 cups of chopped fresh spinach
- Two cloves garlic, minced
- Salt and pepper to taste
- Tortilla chips or bread for serving

Instructions:
1. Set the oven's temperature to 350°F (175°C).
2. Mix the cream cheese, sour cream, mayonnaise, Parmesan cheese, and shredded mozzarella cheese thoroughly in a large mixing dish.
3. Stir well after adding the minced garlic, sliced spinach, and chopped artichoke hearts into the mixture.
4. Salt and pepper to taste is how you should season your food.
5. Spread the mixture in a baking dish.
6. Cook for 20–25 minutes, or until cheese is melted and bubbling.
7. Before serving, take the dish out of the oven and let it cool.
8. Serve hot with tortilla strips or bread.

138. Bacon-Wrapped Dates

Ingredients:

- 12 Medjool dates, pitted
- Six strips of bacon, cut in half
- Toothpicks
- Balsamic glaze

Instructions:

1. The oven should be preheated at 375°F (190°C).
2. There should be a small amount of cheese or almonds inside each pitted date.
3. Each date with filling is wrapped in half a slice of bacon and held together with a toothpick.
4. Place the bacon-wrapped dates on a baking sheet covered in parchment paper.
5. Bake the pork for 15–20 minutes, or until it reaches the desired crispiness.
6. Remove the toothpicks from the bacon-wrapped dates.
7. If using, sprinkle warm food with balsamic glaze.

139. Cucumber Bites

Ingredients:

- One large cucumber
- 4 oz cream cheese, softened
- 2 tbsp. chop fresh dill
- 2 tsp. lemon juice
- Salt and pepper to taste
- Cherry tomatoes, sliced

Instructions:

1. Slice the cucumber into 1/4-inch-thick pieces after cleaning.
2. Mix the cream cheese, dill, lemon juice, salt, and pepper together in a small bowl until everything is well combined.
3. The cream cheese mixture should be spread thinly on each cucumber round.
4. Each round of cucumber should have a cherry tomato slice for presentation.
5. On a serving platter, arrange the cucumber bites.
6. Put the dish in the fridge for at least half an hour to cool down before serving.

140. Chicken Satay Skewers

Ingredients:

- One lb boneless, skinless chicken breasts or thighs cut into thin strips
- 1/2 cups of coconut milk
- 2 tbsp. soy sauce
- 1 tbsp. brown sugar
- 1 tbsp. curry powder
- 1 tsp. ground ginger
- 1 tsp. garlic powder
- Salt and pepper to taste
- Wooden skewers soaked in water for at least 30 minutes
- Peanut sauce

Instructions:

1. Coconut milk, soy sauce, brown sugar, curry powder, ground ginger, garlic powder, salt, and pepper should all be thoroughly combined in a big mixing bowl.
2. Toss the chicken in the coating so that it is evenly coated.
3. It's suggested that you marinate the chicken for at least half an hour in the fridge. Wrap the casserole tightly in plastic.
4. The skillet or grill pan should be preheated to medium-high heat.
5. The wooden skewers should be threaded with chicken pieces.
6. Skewer the chicken and cook it over high heat for 3–4 minutes per side, or until it is no longer pink inside and has a light charred exterior.
7. Before serving, take the food off the grill and let it cool.
8. Serve heated with peanut dipping sauce.

141. Stuffed Mushrooms

Ingredients:

- 24 large mushrooms
- 8 oz cream cheese, softened
- 1/2 cups of grated Parmesan cheese
- Two cloves garlic, minced
- 2 tbsp. chop fresh parsley
- Salt and pepper to taste

Instructions:

1. Set the oven's temperature to 375°F (190°C).
2. Take off the stalks and wash the mushrooms.

3. Mix the cream cheese, grated Parmesan cheese, and minced garlic, and thoroughly chop parsley, salt, and pepper in a small mixing dish.
4. Place a tiny amount of the cream cheese mixture inside each mushroom cap.
5. Prepare a baking sheet with parchment paper and place the stuffed mushrooms on it.
6. To cook the mushrooms in the oven, set the timer for 20–25 minutes.
7. Remove the dish from the oven and let it cool for at least 15 minutes before serving.

142. Chips and Dip

Ingredients:
- One bag of tortilla chips
- 1 cups of sour cream
- 1/2 cups of mayonnaise
- 1 tbsp. dried parsley
- 1 tbsp. dried dill
- 1 tbsp. onion powder
- 1/2 tsp. garlic powder
- Salt and pepper to taste

Instructions:
1. Sour cream, mayonnaise, dried dill, onion powder, garlic powder, salt, and pepper should all be thoroughly combined in a small mixing dish.
2. Put the plastic wrap-covered bowl into the fridge and let the dip chill for at least 30 minutes to let the flavors combine.

3. Arrange the tortilla pieces in an attractive pattern on a serving platter.
4. Put the chips and dip in a dish and serve.

143. Bruschetta Chicken Salad

Ingredients:
- Two boneless, skinless chicken breasts
- 4 cups of mixed greens
- 1 cups of cherry tomatoes, halved
- 1/2 cups of red onion, diced
- 1/4 cups of fresh basil leaves, chop
- Two cloves garlic, minced
- 1 tbsp. balsamic vinegar
- 1 tbsp. olive oil
- Salt and pepper to taste
- Four slices of crusty bread toasted

Instructions:
1. Heat should be warmed to medium-high in the skillet or grill pan.
2. Salt and pepper both sides of the chicken breasts.
3. Grilling the fowl on each side for 5 to 6 minutes should result in thoroughly cooked poultry.
4. Take off the grill, then place the food aside to cool.
5. Add the mixed greens, cherry tomatoes, red onion, and chopped basil
6. in a large mixing bowl.
7. Whisk together the balsamic vinegar, olive oil, salt, and pepper with the minced garlic in a small bowl.

8. The salad should be topped with diced grilled chicken breasts.
9. Dress the salad and toss to combine.
10. The salad should be served with warm bread slices.

144. Greek Salad Skewers

Ingredients:
- Cherry tomatoes
- Cucumber, cut into bite-sized pieces
- Kalamata olives
- Feta cheese cut into bite-sized cubes
- Red onion, cut into bite-sized pieces
- Wooden skewers

For the dressing:

- 1/4 cups of olive oil
- 2 tbsp. red wine vinegar
- 1 tsp. dried oregano
- Salt and pepper to taste

Instructions:
1. To prevent the hardwood skewers from burning while being grilled, soak them in water for at least 30 minutes.
2. Cherry tomatoes, cucumber slices, Kalamata olives, feta cheese cubes, and red onion segments should be threaded onto the wooden skewers.
3. Place the skewers in a line on a serving platter.
4. In a tiny bowl, whisk together the olive oil, red wine vinegar, salt, pepper, and dried oregano.

5. Drizzle the sauce over the skewers after serving.

145. Antipasto Platter

Ingredients:

- Assorted cured meats such as prosciutto, salami, and pepperoni
- Assorted cheeses such as mozzarella, provolone, and parmesan
- Marinated vegetables such as artichoke hearts, roasted red peppers, and olives
- Fresh vegetables such as cherry tomatoes, cucumber slices, and carrot sticks
- Crackers or breadsticks for serving

Instructions:

1. Folding the pieces, arrange the cured meats on a large serving dish in a pleasing pattern.
2. Between the proteins in the dish, arrange the various kinds of cheese.
3. On the platter, distribute the marinated vegetables in an even layer.
4. Add the fresh vegetables and arrange them between the other ingredients on the tray.
5. Serve with appetizers or breadsticks.

146. Meatballs

Ingredients:

- 1 lb ground beef
- 1/2 cups of breadcrumbs
- 1/4 cups of grated parmesan cheese
- 1/4 cups of chopped fresh parsley
- One egg, lightly beaten
- Two cloves garlic, minced
- 1 tsp. salt
- 1/2 tsp. black pepper
- 2 tbsp. olive oil

Instructions:

1. Turn the oven on to 375°F.
2. Ground beef, breadcrumbs, parmesan cheese, chop parsley, beaten egg, minced garlic, salt, and black pepper should all be combined in a sizable mixing dish.
3. Use your hands to combine the materials thoroughly.
4. The mixture can be formed into meatballs between 1 and 2 inches in diameter.
5. Olive oil should be warmed in a large saucepan over medium heat.
6. Turning once, the meatballs need about three minutes in the pan.
7. For optimal results, bake the meatballs for 20 minutes, or until no longer pink in the center.
8. After cooking, set the dish aside to cool to room temperature before serving.

147. Edamame

Ingredients:

- 1 lb edamame in the pod
- 2 tbsp. salt
- Water for boiling

Instructions:

1. Rinse the edamame in a colander, then set it aside.
2. Bring to a boil in a large saucepan enough water to completely cover the edamame.
3. Stir the salt into boiling water to ensure that it dissolves.
4. Cook the edamame for 5-6 minutes in a pot of simmering water.
5. To stop the edamame from boiling, rinse it in cool water, then drain it into a colander.
6. If you'd like, season the edamame with extra salt before serving them in a bowl.

148. Air-Fried Raspberry Brie Bites

Ingredients:

- 1 (8 oz.) round Brie cheese
- 1 (8 oz.) package of phyllo dough, thawed
- 1 cups of raspberry jam
- 1 cups of butter, melted
- 2 tbsp. Honey
- flakey salt to taste

Directions:

1. The brie should be cut into squares between 1.5 and 2 inches wide.
2. Roll out one sheet of phyllo dough vertically on an ample work surface. Before folding the top half of the dough, the lower half should be coated with melted butter.
3. Place one cheese slice in the bottom of the dough's center, 2 inches in from all sides. About 2 tbsp. Raspberry jam should be added to the cheese. Brush the remaining pastry with the melted butter.
4. Then, bring the bottom two inches of dough up and in over the cheese. The leftover dough should be coated with more butter before the filling is gradually rolled upward until it is entirely encased. Put the item in the air fryer after adding extra butter to the top.
5. The oven fryer should be set to 375°F (190°C).
6. 4-5 minutes in the oven at 400 degrees until golden brown. Use a thin honey glaze and some flakes of salt as a finishing touch. Immediately serve.

149. Feta-Spinach Puff Pastry Bites

Ingredients:

- Nonstick cooking spray
- One sheet of frozen puff pastry thawed in the refrigerator
- ¾ cups of mayonnaise
- One (6 oz.) container of crumbled feta cheese
- ½ cups of freshly grated Parmesan cheese

- 1 (10 oz.) package of frozen chop spinach, thawed and drained
- Two cloves garlic, minced
- ¼ tsp. Ground black pepper

Directions:

1. (180 degrees C) Turn the oven on to 375 degrees. A 24-cups of mini muffin tray (or two 12-cups of mini muffin pans) should be sprayed with nonstick cooking spray before use.
2. On a surface that has been lightly floured, a rolling tool is used to shape the cold, thawed puff pastry sheet into a rectangle. Divide the dough into 24 (2 1/2 inch) pieces using a pizza cutter. Puff pastry should be gently pressed into each prepared cups of the small muffin pan before being forked with a fork.
3. Combine the mayonnaise, spinach, garlic, feta cheese, parmesan cheese, and pepper in a dish.
4. Distribute the feta-spinach mixture evenly among the cups of carefully, careful not to overfill them.
5. To get a golden crust and a puffed crust, bake for 15 to 16 minutes.
6. Hold off on serving until the bites have cooled for 5 minutes on a wire rack in the pan.

150. Bisquick Sausage Balls

Ingredients:

- 6 cups of baking mix
- 2 lbs shredded extra-sharp Cheddar cheese
- 1 lb sage-flavored pork sausage at room temperature
- 1 lb hot pork sausage at room temperature

Directions:

1. Put all the parts together.
2. The recommended oven temperature is 300 degrees. At a temperature of 150 C. Spread butter on baking sheets.
3. Combine the baking mix, Cheddar cheese, and hot and sage-flavored pork sausages in a large dish.
4. Form a 1/2-inch thick patty from the sausage mixture and place on the prepared baking sheets.
5. Wait 25-30 minutes in the oven for the outside to brown and the inside to stop looking pink.

28-DAYS MEAL PLAN

Now, it's time for a daily meal plan for you. Let's have a look!

1st WEEK	2nd WEEK	3rd WEEK	4th WEEK
DAY 1	**DAY 8**	**DAY 15**	**DAY 22**
Breakfast: Crescent Breakfast Squares **Lunch:** Slow Cooker Buffalo Chicken Sandwiches **Dinner:** Grilled Shrimp Skewers with Mango Salsa	**Breakfast:** Ham and Cheese Breakfast Casserole **Lunch:** Caldo de Pollo **Dinner:** Stuffed Peppers	**Breakfast:** Vermicelli Noodle Bowl **Lunch:** Traditional Gyros **Dinner:** Slow Cooker Beef Stew	**Breakfast:** Super Easy Egg Casserole **Lunch:** Creamy Tomato Soup with Grilled Cheese Sandwiches **Dinner:** Tacos al Pastor
DAY 2	**DAY 9**	**DAY 16**	**DAY 23**
Breakfast: Muesli **Lunch:** Taco Bell Seasoning Copycat **Dinner:** Baked Ziti with Sausage and Ricotta	**Breakfast:** Oatmeal Soda Bread **Lunch:** Philly Steak Sandwich **Dinner:** Beef and Broccoli Stir-Fry	**Breakfast:** Yogurt Parfait with Granola and Fruit **Lunch:** Three Bean Salad **Dinner:** Lasagna Flatbread	**Breakfast:** Spinach and Feta Omelette **Lunch:** Ukrainian Red Borscht Soup **Dinner:** One-Pot Beef Stew
DAY 3	**DAY 10**	**DAY 17**	**DAY 24**
Breakfast: Irish Soda Bread **Lunch:** Sloppy Joes **Dinner:** Beef and Mushroom Stroganoff	**Breakfast:** Biscuits and Gravy **Lunch:** Easy French Dip Sandwiches **Dinner:** Eggplant Parmesan	**Breakfast:** Fluffy French Toast **Lunch:** Broccoli Cheese Soup **Dinner:** Stout-Braised Lamb Shanks	**Breakfast:** Breakfast Burrito **Lunch:** Delicious Egg Salad for Sandwiches **Dinner:** Grilled Steak with Chimichurri Sauce

DAY 4	DAY 11	DAY 18	DAY 25
Breakfast: Breakfast Strata with Sausage and Spinach **Lunch:** Pasta Salad **Dinner:** Black Bean and Corn Quesadillas	**Breakfast:** Greek Yogurt Waffles **Lunch:** Zesty Quinoa Salad **Dinner:** Spicy Sausage and Vegetable Skillet	**Breakfast:** Delicious Egg Salad for Sandwiches **Lunch:** Homemade Corn Dogs **Dinner:** Mississippi Chicken	**Breakfast:** Quiche Lorraine **Lunch:** Best Cream of Broccoli Soup **Dinner:** Spaghetti Bolognese

DAY 5	DAY 12	DAY 19	DAY 26
Breakfast: Crème Brûlée French Toast **Lunch:** Reuben Sandwich **Dinner:** Grilled Teriyaki Chicken Skewers	**Breakfast:** Breakfast Hash with Sweet Potatoes and Sausage **Lunch:** Best Ramen Noodle Salad **Dinner:** Shrimp Scampi	**Breakfast:** Scrambled Egg Muffin Cups **Lunch:** Fresh Tomato Soup **Dinner:** Baked Salmon with Lemon and Herbs	**Breakfast:** Bacon and Egg Breakfast Pizza **Lunch:** Old Fashioned Potato Salad **Dinner:** Vegetable Stir-Fry

DAY 6	DAY 13	DAY 20	DAY 27
Breakfast: Sweet French Toast **Lunch:** Super-Delicious Zuppa Toscana **Dinner:** Chicken Tikka Masala	**Breakfast:** Breakfast Quesadilla **Lunch:** Best Bean Salad **Dinner:** Slow Cooker Texas Pulled Pork	**Breakfast:** Classic Eggs Benedict **Lunch:** Best Chicken Salad **Dinner:** Chicken Fajitas	**Breakfast:** Vermicelli Noodle Bowl **Lunch:** Curried Egg Sandwiches **Dinner:** Chicken Caesar Salad

DAY 7	DAY 14	DAY 21	DAY 28
Breakfast: Shakshuka **Lunch**: Baked Potato Soup **Dinner**: Ratatouille	**Breakfast**: Garlic Bread Spread **Lunch**: Simple Pasta Salad **Dinner**: Homemade Mac and Cheese	**Breakfast**: Sausage and Egg Breakfast Sandwich **Lunch**: Pasta Salad with Homemade Dressing **Dinner**: Corned Beef Roast	**Breakfast**: Breakfast Hash with Sweet Potatoes and Sausage **Lunch**: Best Ramen Noodle Salad **Dinner**: Shrimp Scampi

Conclusion

In conclusion, "The Ulcerative Colitis Cookbook" is a valuable resource for individuals with ulcerative colitis. The cookbook provides delicious recipes that are easy to prepare and gentle on the digestive system, making it easier for individuals with this condition to maintain a healthy diet.

The cookbook includes breakfast, lunch, dinner, and snack recipes, focusing on low-fibre, low-fat, and low-residue ingredients. The book also provides valuable information on ulcerative colitis, including its symptoms, causes, and management.

Overall, "The Ulcerative Colitis Cookbook" is helpful for anyone looking to manage ulcerative colitis through dietary changes. The recipes are nutritious, easy to digest, tasty and satisfying. It is a highly recommended resource for individuals with ulcerative colitis and their loved ones.